PRAISE FOR
TRANSFORMING THE SHAME TRIANGLE

"*Transforming the Shame Triangle* presents an extremely helpful model for working with the internal dynamics that keep us caught in cycles of shame and suffering, as well as clarifying understandings of the external systems and structures which generate such dynamics. Weaving together multiple wisdoms and practices in an accessible and engaging way, Jessica and David help us to honour the deeply plural nature of ourselves, and help all find their ways towards love and liberation."
—Meg-John Barker, author of the *Plural Selves* zines and *Rewriting the Rules*

"Jessica Fern and David Cooley have made a giant leap in moving us forward in developing new and effective healing modalities. They truly deliver the complete package, for clinicians and for the rest of us. Don't be distracted by their brilliant synthesis of many psychotherapeutic theories. They take that to the next level and come through with the praxis, putting theory into practice. This book takes that robust analysis and then provides step-by-step instructions for utilizing their innovative tools for healing trauma and breaking free from life-long beliefs and patterns of behavior."
—Kathy Labriola, nurse, counselor and author of *The Polyamory Breakup Book*

"Fern and Cooley have done a beautiful job making the complex processes of shame and self-love accessible and nuanced. This book is a practical roadmap for anyone who wants to bridge the gap between psychological insight and real-world application, offering both deeper understanding of how we get trapped in shame-fuelled patterns and actionable steps toward genuine self-acceptance. Their framework provides hope without over-simplification, making meaningful personal transformation feel genuinely achievable."
—Shadeen Francis, relationship and family therapist

"Shame is a prevailing issue in people's psychology and leads to a multitude of problems in relationships. In this book, Jessica Fern and David Cooley provide incredibly helpful tools in aiding clinicians and clients in working through and managing shame. I would highly recommend *Transforming the Shame Triangle* for anyone looking to increase their understanding of how to use parts work to manage emotions and address problems."
—Tamara Pincus, licensed clinical social worker, sex therapist and co-author of *It's Called Polyamory*

"An absolute must-read for anyone caught in the endless chase to 'be better,' *Transforming the Shame Triangle* breaks us free from painful cycles of compulsive self-improvement, affirming that self-love isn't a reward we earn by being better—it's already here, ready to emerge when we hold the parts of ourselves we've been taught to hide. Step by step, Jessica Fern and David Cooley teach us how. With elegant research, relatable stories and practical exercises, they provide a deceptively simple, memorable framework that belongs on the bookshelf of every therapist, coach, educator and self-healer."
—Hailey Magee, author of *Stop People Pleasing and Find Your Power*

**Transforming
the Shame
Triangle**

ALSO BY JESSICA FERN AND DAVID COOLEY

Polywise: A Deeper Dive into Navigating Open Relationships

ALSO BY JESSICA FERN

Polysecure: Attachment, Trauma and Consensual Nonmonogamy

The Polysecure Workbook: Healing Your Attachment and Creating Security in Loving Relationships

TRANSFORMING THE SHAME TRIANGLE

From Shame to Love Using Parts Work

Jessica Fern and David Cooley

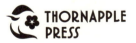
THORNAPPLE PRESS

Transforming the Shame Triangle
From Shame to Love Using Parts Work
Copyright ©2025 by Jessica Fern and David Cooley

All rights reserved. No part of this book may be used or reproduced in any manner whatsoever without written permission from the publisher except in the case of brief quotations in critical articles and reviews.

NO AI TRAINING: Without in any way limiting the author's and publisher's exclusive rights under copyright, any use of this publication to "train" generative artificial intelligence (AI) technologies to generate text is expressly prohibited. The publisher reserves all rights to license uses of this work for generative AI training and development of machine learning language models.

Thornapple Press
300 – 722 Cormorant Street
Victoria, BC V8W 1P8 Canada
press@thornapplepress.ca

EU Authorised Representative: Easy Access System Europe -
Mustamäe tee 50, 10621 Tallinn, Estonia, gpsr.requests@easproject.com

Our business offices are located on the traditional, ancestral and unceded territories of the lək̓ʷəŋən and W̱SÁNEĆ peoples. We return a percentage of company profits to the original stewards of this land through South Island Reciprocity Trust.

Thornapple Press is a brand of Talk Science to Me Communications Inc. Talk Science is a WBE Canada Certified Women Business Enterprise, a CGLCC Certified 2SLGBTQI+-owned business, and a Certified Living Wage Employer.

 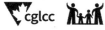

Cover and interior design by Jeffrey Werner
Substantive editing by Andrea Zanin
Copy-editing by Heather van der Hoop
Proofreading by Alison Whyte
Index by Siusan Moffat

Library and Archives Canada Cataloging-In-Publication Data
Title: Transforming the shame triangle : from shame to love using parts work / Jessican Fern and David Cooley.
Names: Fern, Jessica, author. | Cooley, David (Restorative justice facilitator), author.
Description: Includes bibliographical references and index.
Identifiers: Canadiana (print) 20250226537 | Canadiana (ebook) 20250227738 | ISBN 9781990869709 (softcover) | ISBN 9781990869914 (PDF) | ISBN 9781990869716 (EPUB)
Subjects: LCSH: Shame. | LCSH: Self-acceptance. | LCSH: Systemic therapy (Family therapy) | LCSH: Narrative therapy.
Classification: LCC BF575.S45 F47 2025 | DDC 152.4/4—dc23

10 9 8 7 6 5 4 3 2 1

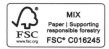

Printed and bound in Canada by Friesens.

CONTENTS

Acknowledgments	vii
Introduction	1
My Journey to Parts Work	6
About Us: Jess and Dave	29
A Note on Shame Versus shame	35
Book Overview	35
Chapter 1: The Drama Triangle	39
Why So Much Drama?	45
Who Starts the Triangle?	53
Getting Off the Drama Triangle	56
Chapter 2: Getting to Know Your Shame Triangle	67
The Inner Critic	68
Shame	78
Escapers	88
How Your Shame Triangle Parts Instigate Each Other	97
Chapter 3: Shame Triangle Origins and Triggers	99
Where Does the Shame Triangle Come From?	99
Recognizing Internalization	108
Shame Triangle Triggers	110
The Trouble with Positive Events	113
Chapter 4: The Self	119
The Self in IFS	123
Exercises for Cultivating Self-Connection	134
Chapter 5: Becoming Self-Centered in Body, Heart and Mind	149
The Self-Centered Model	152
The Body Center	155
The Heart Center	160
The Mind Center	165
Evaluating Your Three Centers	169
Integration and Reflection: Bringing the Three Centers into Balance	174

Chapter 6: Dialoguing with Your Parts	177
The Absent but Implicit	179
A Few Common Concerns Before You Begin	183
The Transformation Process	186
Transforming the Inner Critic	187
Transforming Shame	195
Transforming Escapers	202
Chapter 7: The Shame Triangle and the Body	209
The Shame Triangle and Nervous System Survival Responses	210
The Inner Critic and the Fight Response Turned Inward	211
Shame and the Freeze Response	213
Escapers and the Four F's	215
Regulating the Four F Responses of the Nervous System	218
Listening to the Body's Wisdom	229
Chapter 8: The Shame Triangle and the Heart	233
Heart Center Exercises	244
Chapter 9: The Shame Triangle and the Mind	255
Shame Triangle Mindsets	256
Self-Led Mindsets	262
Shift Your Mindset Prompts	271
The R's of Releasing Beliefs and Resonating with New Ones	274
Chapter 10: When Your Shame Triangle Isn't Yours	281
Exercises	289
Chapter 11: Bringing Our Shame Triangle Parts Together into the Self-Love Triangle	305
Repair Processes	308
Create Your Own Ritual	316
Conclusion	319
Appendix	323
EASE Process for Working with Your Parts	323
References	327
Index	331

ACKNOWLEDGMENTS

This book is built on the ideas, practices and wisdom of many who have come before us. We're grateful to the teachers, thought leaders and communities whose work laid the foundation for our own. We especially want to acknowledge the influence of Internal Family Systems (IFS) and narrative therapy, and the guidance of our Buddhist and shamanic teachers. These traditions and frameworks have shaped the roots of this book and the spirit in which it was written.

A heartfelt thank you to Julia Taylor for your generous insights and supportive conversations that helped sharpen our somatic lens, especially in the sections on the body and nervous system. Your contributions made this work stronger and more embodied.

To Jessica McDuffee—thank you for inviting me (Jessica) to awaken together and for walking this path side by side. Our shared journey sessions have brought invaluable insight into these ideas, and your willingness to experiment and test out these practices has truly elevated the work.

Nai Kaya—we see you! Your magic and medicine helped shape key features of the Self-centered model, and your presence has been felt in more ways than one. Thank you for being an amazing cheerleader throughout this whole process. Your support, insight and enthusiasm have meant the world to us.

We are also grateful to Thornapple Press for supporting this book into being. Thank you to Eve, Hazel, Andrea, Heather and Jeff for your editorial guidance and thoughtful feedback. Thanks as well to our additional readers, whose perspectives helped refine the final shape of this work.

And to Diego—thank you for your patience with two parents writing a book on top of working full time. Although we're pretty sure you didn't mind the extra screen time ;)

INTRODUCTION

As I clicked "End Meeting" on my screen, the familiar silence of my office settled in. The last video session of the day with a therapy client had just wrapped up. I exhaled, sinking into my chair, but despite the day winding down, I felt an internal tug-of-war revving up. My eyes jumped to the unread emails in my inbox. The diligent taskmaster in me urged me to tackle them now. But the mother part of me wanted nothing more than to check in with my son, to hear about his day. A glance at my phone revealed a cascade of notifications—my sister sending funny cat GIFs, my mom needing input on family logistics, my partner leaving a voice memo, a friend reaching out with difficult news. The sister, daughter, partner and friend in me all felt the pull to respond immediately.

And yet, there was another voice—one reminding me that before I turned outward again, I needed to pause and reconnect within. After a day of holding space for others, I longed to feel grounded first in myself, then with my son, and texts could come after. As for the emails, I found myself wishing for an assistant or the ability to freeze time so I could tackle them without sacrificing my personal needs or family time, knowing they'd be better handled with fresh eyes in the morning.

All these competing needs reminded me how often I think about myself in terms of parts. By "parts," I mean the different aspects of myself, each with its own concerns, priorities and desires, creating the amalgam that is me. The concept of me as a whole person—Jessica—is made up not of one facet, but many. The nurturer who loves making breakfast for others. The professional seeking purpose. The dreamer lost in ideas. The lover desiring intimacy. The loyal friend, the quiet introvert, the inner child who still fears the dark. And the sassy teenager who is fiercely independent—just to name a few.

At any given moment, I find myself asking: Which part of me is speaking right now? Which part is feeling this emotion? Is it a protective part? A wounded part? A wise part? When I'm talking with a friend, which part of me is showing up? The part that wants to sound smart? The part that genuinely seeks connection? Or the part that is people-pleasing? The same goes for my relationship—what parts of my partner do I feel safe with, drawn to or frustrated by? What parts of me support our relationship, and which get in the way?

If you're already familiar with the idea of having different inner parts, great—you're with me so far. For those new to this concept, you might not already think of yourself as having multiple inner parts per se, but you probably recognize having different sides to who you are: a serious side in some situations, a playful side in others, or a competitive side when the stakes are high. You might relate to feeling torn between going out or staying home, between one part that feels obligated to show up and another that just wants to rest. Similarly, you might experience a conflict between one part that's committed to a healthy lifestyle and another that craves indulgence.

I didn't always think this way. Like many people, I used to believe I had one "true self"—a single, unified identity, something unchanging and stable at the core of who I was. Many of us are taught this from an early age. We hear phrases like "be yourself" or "find your true self," as if there's one definitive version of us waiting to be uncovered. We're conditioned to think of ourselves as a singular "I," and when we experience contradictions—one part of us wanting connection while another pulls away, one part craving risk while another prefers caution—we assume we're just indecisive or inconsistent, or there's something wrong with us. But what if this inner push and pull isn't a flaw, but a fundamental truth of how our minds work? What if these contradictions aren't mistakes to be corrected, but evidence of something essential—something natural?

The idea that we are made up of multiple parts isn't new. Philosophers, psychologists and people in various spiritual traditions have long explored the multiplicity of the human mind. Plato described the soul as having distinct aspects, each with different motivations and desires—reason, spirit and appetite—all vying for control. Descartes later proposed that the mind and body were separate yet intertwined, fueling centuries of debate about what constitutes a person's true essence. Many religious traditions emphasize a duality between body and spirit, while others suggest that even the soul itself can fragment and require reintegration.

Despite these perspectives, modern culture conditions us to believe in a singular self. We're taught to fit into neat categories—introvert or extrovert, thinker or feeler, organized or messy, a hugger or not. But if you've ever felt torn between responsibility and desire, logic and emotion, what you want and what you feel you *should* do, you've already encountered the truth that we are not as singular as we assume. This realization can be confusing because even when we recognize different aspects of ourselves, we're often taught to see them as problems rather than natural parts of being human.

For example, hearing about "parts" may bring to mind narratives like that of Dr. Jekyll and Mr. Hyde or film tropes about people with multiple personalities, which can reinforce fears that having different sides makes us unstable, disorganized or dangerous. The underlying message is that if you don't feel entirely consistent all the time, something must be wrong with you. While extreme fragmentation, such as dissociative identity disorder,* exists and can be distressing, it represents a very specific and uncommon experience in which parts become so separated that people may lose time or have no awareness

---

* Previously known as multiple personality disorder.

of shifting from one part to another. For most people, however, even strong internal conflicts or shifts in mood happen with some degree of awareness and memory. Parts within our human psychology exist on a broad and relatable spectrum of intensity. Feeling reactive, torn or overwhelmed by different internal voices is not a sign of pathology—it's a reflection of our complexity, and a sign that there's more going on inside us than we've been taught to see. Having internal parts is not a disorder—it's a normal and intelligent aspect of being human. Our parts aren't a problem; they are a reflection of our depth, adaptability and ability to function, love, create and grow.

That said, even within the normal range of human experience, some parts make life difficult. They may sabotage us, carry trauma, hold us back from opportunities, push away loved ones, get defensive, dwell in shame or engage in self-destructive behaviors. Because many of these parts first formed when we were children or adolescents, they often continue to think and react with the level of emotional and cognitive development we had at that earlier time. In essence, they're trying to run our adult lives with a child's logic, which is why they're often overwhelmed, impulsive or reactive—even when they have the best of intentions. If left unexamined, they can drive us toward actions we later regret, distort how we see ourselves and create roadblocks in our relationships. The key isn't to fear or reject them, but to develop a new kind of relationship with them.

This book is about change—real and lasting change. It is a guide for loving the parts of yourself that may seem the most unlovable and overwhelming, and transforming them into allies instead of enemies. More specifically, this book explores the three particular parts I believe create the greatest barriers to psychological and spiritual health. I call them the Shame Triangle, an internalized version of the Drama Triangle (more on that later). These three parts are:

- **The Inner Critic**: the voice in our head that judges, belittles and finds fault, holding us to impossible standards or telling us we're never enough.

- **Shame**: the part that feels like something is fundamentally wrong or broken inside you. It says if people really saw you, they'd turn away. It makes you shrink, hide and silence yourself to avoid the risk of rejection.
- **The Escaper**: the part (or parts) that copes with self-criticism and shame by numbing, avoiding or distracting through overworking, overperforming, withdrawing or other forms of escapism.

Together, these parts create a cycle of self-judgment, shame and avoidance—one that can quite literally take over our entire lives. They shape how we see ourselves, dictate the risks we take and the dreams we abandon, and limit the love and connection we allow ourselves to give and receive. This inner triangle erodes our confidence, fuels self-sabotage and convinces us we are fundamentally unworthy. It keeps us stuck, disconnected and unable to fully engage with the life we long for.

I wish I could say I was exaggerating, but I'm not.

But that cycle doesn't have to define us. These parts, as overwhelming as they might seem, are not who we are at our core. Just as these parts hold us back, they also hold the key to our transformation. And when we learn how to work with them—rather than being controlled by them—we open the door to something far greater: freedom. Real, lasting freedom to live, love and express ourselves without the weight of constant self-judgment and fear.

Parts work helps unify these different aspects of our inner world by building a conscious, supportive relationship between them. It allows us to acknowledge their needs, address their fears, update their beliefs and guide them toward healthier roles. Through this process of working with our many parts, we can develop a clearer, stronger sense of Self. In the pages ahead, we'll begin this journey—not by fighting our parts, but by using parts work to understand them, transform them and step into a new way of being.

My Journey to Parts Work

Before we get into transforming the Shame Triangle, I want to share how I arrived at this work. I think the context will help. This shift didn't happen overnight. I spent years immersed in different models of psychology, conflict resolution and spiritual practice, each offering insights that resonated deeply but still left gaps I struggled to reconcile. I was searching for something cohesive, something that could integrate all these perspectives into a framework that truly made sense of both the inner and outer conflicts we face. I wanted to feel as effective as possible in what I was offering to others and, many times, I was simply trying to make sense of my own inner world.

My first exposure to the idea that we are made up of different internal forces was in a high school Intro to Psychology class with Freud's model of the psyche. His concept of the id, ego and superego challenged my assumption that I was a singular self. Instead, Freud framed the mind as a battleground—one part seeking pleasure and impulse (id), another trying to enforce morality and social rules (superego), and the ego left to mediate between them. While I never fully aligned with Freud's ideas, the seed was planted that we are made up of multiple, sometimes conflicting, inner forces.

As in most introductory psychology classes, after Freud came Jung. His work expanded my understanding, introducing the idea that we carry universal archetypes within us—timeless roles like the Hero, who embarks on the journey of discovery; the Persona, who upholds the mask we present to the world; the Shadow, which embodies our hidden fears and desires; and the Anima and Animus, which represent inner feminine and masculine energies. These weren't just abstract ideas for me. As a kid with a rocky home life, the notion that I might tap into these archetypal sources of strength gave me hope for creating my own change. If my external circumstances were unstable, maybe I could cultivate internal strengths to help me navigate them. Jung's framework gave me a sense of agency—the idea that I wasn't just reacting to life, but had an entire cast of inner characters who could support me in different ways.

Several years later, my continued study of archetypes led me to Caroline Myss, who offered a psycho-spiritual lens on Jung's work. Myss posits that within the vast spectrum of potential archetypes—the Mother, Mystic, Networker, Saboteur, Engineer, Trickster, Poet, Athlete and many more—we each embody and express twelve primary archetypal patterns. These twelve form the unique core of our personalities, much like how a painter selects a specific palette from an endless array of colors to create a signature piece, or how our names, though composed of only a handful of letters from the alphabet, come together to form something distinct and personal to us.

What stood out to me most was Myss's emphasis on the light and shadow within each archetype. The King archetype, for instance, can be a wise and benevolent leader or an entitled ruler who seeks to dominate through absolute control. The Addict's light side channels intense desire into self-awareness, devotion and healthy choices, while its shadow succumbs to destructive cravings. The Rebel can challenge injustice and enact meaningful change, or it can resist authority out of resentment. If we assume some archetypes are inherently good and others bad, we may believe that certain ones set us up for failure while others guarantee success. But that's a false premise. It's not about which archetypes we have—it's about how they show up. All parts carry both potential and peril.

Instead of viewing certain aspects of ourselves as flaws to overcome, Myss's work showed me that even the more difficult or unwanted parts have the potential to serve us in healthier ways. We can consciously support our archetypes in expressing their light rather than their shadow. That simple but powerful shift—seeing all parts as capable of harm or growth—would later become essential to my work in parts psychology.

Still, something was missing. While Jung and Myss helped me understand *who* lived inside me, I didn't yet have a way of understanding *how* these parts interacted. That understanding came when I began training in conflict resolution and discovered the Drama Triangle.

The Drama Triangle

Created by psychiatrist Stephen Karpman in the late 1960s, this psychological and social model of human interaction outlines three archetypal roles: the Victim, the Persecutor and the Rescuer. The Persecutor criticizes, blames or controls; the Victim feels powerless or mistreated; and the Rescuer rushes in to help, often without being asked, while neglecting their own needs. It's the classic hero-villain-victim storyline, playing out in everyday life. These three parts represent the positions we unconsciously assume or are thrust into during conflict situations; we cast ourselves and others into certain roles, resulting in dynamics that create discord, damage, disappointment and of course, drama.

When Karpman used the term "drama," he referred to the intense, often exaggerated emotional interactions that escalate tension like scenes in a theatrical performance, overshadowing genuine connection and resolution. Though we rarely intend to be dramatic, we may often find ourselves slipping into these roles, perpetuating conflict rather than fostering constructive communication. In the vast landscape of personal development tools, I have found few concepts that have the power to illuminate the dynamics of personal interactions quite like the Drama Triangle—in the bedroom, the living room, the boardroom and all the way to the international stage.

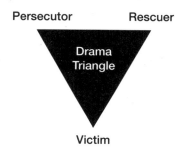

These ideas gave me a new lens on my relationships, helping me better understand both long-standing dysfunctional dynamics and the smaller, everyday interactions that felt unsatisfying. For the first time, I could recognize how different parts of myself and others shaped our conflicts. Instead of labeling someone else or even myself as "difficult" or "toxic," I began to see how we all unconsciously fall into these roles that keep conflict alive. Later, when I shared these insights with clients and workshop participants, they also found new ways to enrich their relationships by either circumventing the Drama Triangle or establishing necessary boundaries with those unwilling to disengage from it. This was a breakthrough, but even with that clarity, something still wasn't clicking. I understood the roles, but I still felt stuck inside them—like the story had already been written, and I was just playing out a script. That's when narrative therapy entered the picture.

Narrative Practice: Naming the Problem, Not Becoming the Problem

My next significant leap in understanding and working with parts came through the lens of poststructuralist narrative theory. During my graduate studies, I was introduced to the idea that our lives are not just a series of objective events, but that we make meaning through the stories we tell about them. Narrative theory challenges the assumption that reality is something objective waiting to be discovered. Instead, it posits that reality is largely constructed—shaped not only by our individual interpretations, but by the cultural, familial and societal narratives we inherit. These stories are not personal inventions; they are absorbed from the world around us, passed down through family beliefs, social norms, systemic power structures and lived experience. From an early age, we internalize messages about who we are supposed to be—what success looks like, what makes us lovable and what is considered worthy or shameful. Some of these narratives empower us. Others confine us, creating invisible limits on our identity and how we show up in the world. At the heart of narrative practice is the idea that we are multi-storied beings. Our identities are not singular or static, but built from many different experiences. Yet when we struggle—emotionally, relationally or professionally—we tend to collapse into one rigid narrative. Michael White and David Epston, the founders of narrative therapy, called this a problem-saturated story (1990). In this state, one storyline—usually a painful or limiting one—overshadows everything else, shaping how we see ourselves, others and what we believe is possible.

A parent who misses their child's performance may conclude, *I'm a terrible parent*, dismissing all the ways they show up with love and care. A professional who makes a mistake at work may spiral into thoughts like *I'm incompetent*, ignoring years of successful contributions. A partner who hears their loved one ask for more connection may interpret it as *Nothing I do is ever enough*, missing the deeper invitation to be closer.

But our problem-saturated stories are not objective truths—they are interpretations. And interpretations can be questioned, revised and rewritten. This is one of the most powerful lessons of narrative practice: the ability to re-author our own lives. Through a wider lens, we can begin to shift from problem-saturated stories to *preferred* stories—ones that hold the full complexity of who we are. That same parent who tells themselves *I'm a terrible parent* can begin to see a more complete picture: They may feel disappointed about missing an event, but they can also recognize the many ways they support and love their child. The employee who fears *I'm incompetent* can acknowledge their mistake while also remembering their skills, growth and past successes. The partner who hears *Nothing I do is ever enough* can start to recognize the request for what it is—not a condemnation, but an opportunity for deeper connection. These shifts don't erase hardship, but they allow us to see ourselves with more nuance, honesty and balance.

When we struggle—whether within ourselves or in our relationships—we often believe the problem is either inside us or intrinsic to someone else. We confuse the presence of a problem with the truth of who we are, thinking things like *I'm broken* or *They'll never change*. Statements like these collapse our entire identity into the struggle—we're not just experiencing anxiety, we *are* anxious; not just feeling shame, we *are* pathetic. This totalizing language leaves no room for complexity or movement. But narrative practice invites us to see problems differently: not as issues located inside a person, but as external forces, shaped by the stories we have internalized, often without realizing it.

In narrative therapy, a technique called externalization involves separating the problem from the person so we can see the issue as something outside of us, not a reflection of who we are. Externalization helps us step back and ask different questions—ones that place the problem outside of us, while still honoring the influence it has. Instead of thinking *I am pathetic*, we can ask, *How does this judgment affect the way I see myself or others?* Instead of believing *I am anxious*, we can think, *Anxiety is showing up right now, trying to take control*. These kinds of questions can help us see that we are not the problem—we have a relationship with the problem. And relationships can change.

I was amazed at how effective—and surprisingly playful—this technique could be. Clients who had spent years weighed down by self-judgment suddenly engaged with their struggles in an entirely new way. One client externalized their anxious part as The Worry Monster, a frantic creature constantly warning of disaster. Another named their procrastination part Maybe Later, recognizing how it held them back. A client struggling in her marriage jokingly called one of their patterns Princess Poopy Pants (her words, not mine). These names weren't just silly—they created enough emotional distance for people to step back, see their patterns clearly and start shifting them. Externalization isn't about minimizing our struggles. It's about seeing them as separate from who we are—giving us the space to challenge them, question them and ultimately, transform them. Yet even as I worked on owning my stories and externalizing my problems, I still wrestled with something deeper. Naming and separating from problem-saturated stories helped, but it also left me with a lingering question: Who was doing the noticing? If I could step back and observe my thoughts, emotions and behaviors as parts, what was the part that was watching? What remained when I externalized everything?

My Spiritual Roots and Cross-Cultural Influences

While psychological theories shaped my understanding of the human mind, my perspective was equally shaped by the spiritual traditions and cultural landscapes I was immersed in. I grew up in Brooklyn, New York, in a family that was itself a cultural tapestry. My relatives came from different parts of Eastern and Western Europe, so I never identified with a singular ethnicity but rather as a "mutt" of many immigrant lineages—Irish, English, Italian and Jewish.

At the same time, I was raised in a predominantly Black neighborhood where I was one of the few white kids in my school and on my block. My world was shaped by the rhythms, richness and realities of people whose backgrounds were different from my own. My block was home to stores and restaurants owned by people who had immigrated from all over the world. This exposure to so many cultural spaces and perspectives taught me that there are countless ways to see and engage with the world. I'm grateful for this experience on one hand—but on the other, I never experienced a singular cultural home I could settle into or rely on. Like anyone, I was shaped by my surroundings, and in my case, that meant growing up in one of the most diverse melting pots in the world.

My family practiced both Judaism and Catholicism, but even as a child, I resisted many of the patriarchal structures and injustices I saw in both traditions. Instead, I found myself drawn to the alternative spiritual influences around me—ones that felt more inclusive, practical and alive. My Cuban Catholic godmother practiced a mix of new age spirituality, inner healing and energy work. My Italian American stepfather, who practiced kung fu, introduced me to martial arts and yoga philosophy. Their teachings weren't rooted in rigid doctrines but in lived experience, in ways of relating to the world that felt more expansive and empowering.

Because of New York City's diversity, I had far more exposure to Eastern spiritual traditions than to the indigenous, pagan or shamanic traditions of my own European ancestry. In the 1990s and 2000s, Buddhist temples, yoga centers and shamanic circles from Latin America and Tibet were relatively accessible, while the spiritual traditions of my ancestors were harder to find or reclaim. If they still existed, I had no direct access to them, and even today, reconnecting with them remains a complex and ongoing process.

While I've studied with a range of teachers and traditions, it's also been important to discern which teachers truly embodied the integrity of what they were teaching. I've learned deeply from some and had to step away from others when their behavior or use of power did not align with the teachings they espoused. Over time, I've had to clarify what it means to have a direct relationship with spirituality and a greater intelligence, rather than outsourcing that connection to external authorities. My understanding of whiteness has also evolved—and continues to evolve. While I've often felt disconnected from a clear cultural lineage, I also recognize that being seen and treated as white comes with a specific set of privileges in the United States—privileges that have undeniably shaped my experience, whether or not I consciously claimed or felt aligned with them.

Feeling like a spiritual orphan awakened the seeker in me. If I couldn't find the traditions of my ancestors, I would turn to what was available. I studied at the Integral Yoga Institute with my stepfather. In college, I traveled to Thailand to explore Theravada Buddhism, later deepening my Vipassana meditation practice at the Insight Meditation Society in the United States. I spent years immersed in Tibetan Buddhism and Dzogchen through various centers in Colorado. These Buddhist teachings—particularly their emphasis on impermanence, nonattachment and the constructed nature of self—deepened my understanding of identity as something fluid rather than fixed.

At the same time, I studied different shamanic practices, from core and neo-shamanism to more specific teachings from Tibetan shamanism and the Inka and Q'ero traditions of Peru. I explored these practices through formal training, study groups, plant medicines and guided experiences. I've studied mindfulness for over twenty-five years and shamanic traditions for over twenty and only in the last few years have I begun to access Celtic shamanism and the Euro-indigenous teachings that connect to my own ancestry.

As my studies deepened, so did my awareness of cultural appropriation: how Westerners often borrow from non-Western spiritual traditions without fully respecting their origins or the people who have preserved them for generations. I strive to be conscientious about this dynamic. Whenever possible, I've studied directly with teachers who explicitly choose to share their traditions with Western students, or I've learned from Western teachers with blessings and formal training from their lineage holders. Still, I understand that these conversations are far from resolved. Many Indigenous people and teachers have voiced concerns about misrepresentation, commodification and lack of accountability within these cross-cultural exchanges. I recognize that much of what I've encountered may be a "copy of a copy"—adapted, diluted or disconnected from its roots, even when offered with the best intentions.

For these reasons, I don't claim to represent any tradition in its original form. I see myself as a student—someone who has learned from many streams, including those that have been altered through Western transmission. The practices I share are filtered through my own experience and study, not presented as pure expressions of the cultures they came from. I share these reflections because my background—influenced by a mix of cultural exposure and a lack of direct ancestral connection—inevitably shaped my approach to healing and transformation. Just as psychology influenced my understanding of inner work, so too did these diverse spiritual teachings. You'll notice their influence woven throughout this book—not as a requirement for belief, but as perspectives that have shaped how I understand change, growth and what it means to truly transform.

The Challenge of Bringing These Streams Together

So far, I have introduced several foundational concepts that set the direction for our exploration in this book. Each of these frameworks provided me with invaluable insight into personal and relational growth, yet I often grappled with how to harmonize them. While mindfulness and meditation cultivated presence, and shamanic practices offered ritual and a felt sense of connection to ancestors and the larger universe, they didn't seamlessly integrate with the psychological models I was trained in. Buddhism emphasized witnessing and detachment, while psychology emphasized engagement and change. They often felt like separate silos—spirituality on one side, psychology on the other—and I needed a way to bridge the gaps between them.

Moreover, while understanding the multiplicity of self was enlightening, intellectual insight alone didn't automatically lead to lasting shifts. Instead of achieving inner harmony, I often found myself caught in power struggles between different parts—one side pushing for healing, another resisting, another skeptical of the whole process. To navigate this tension, I explored therapeutic practices like eye movement desensitization and reprocessing (EMDR), somatic experiencing therapy, attachment therapy, integral theory and energy healing. Each offered valuable tools—ways to process trauma, regulate emotions and deepen self-awareness. But I was still searching for something that could fully integrate these insights into a framework that felt cohesive, both for myself and for the people I worked with.

Enter Internal Family Systems

After completing my graduate studies and spending several years immersed in parts work, I discovered Internal Family Systems (IFS), which felt like uncovering the Rosetta Stone for everything I had been searching for. Unlike other therapeutic models that saw some parts as pathological or dysfunctional, IFS presented a radically different view: All parts, no matter how extreme or painful, have a positive intention. Developed by Richard Schwartz (1995, 2021), IFS is based on the idea that the mind isn't a singular entity but a system of distinct subpersonalities, or "parts." Just like a family consists of different members, our inner world is made up of different parts—some wounded, some protective, and others embodying creativity, joy and other wonderful qualities. A core principle of IFS is that these parts aren't obstacles to be eliminated, but aspects of us that, when understood, can become valuable resources.

A harsh part may be trying to protect us from failure. An anxious part may believe it's keeping us safe. A numbing part might be trying to shield us from pain. These roles are not inherent; they emerge in response to trauma, difficult life experiences, and cultural or familial conditioning. The goal of IFS is not to squash or control these parts but to help them release their extreme roles, uncover their positive intentions, unburden their wounds and adopt more adaptive ways to support us.

At the center of this process is the Self: a core presence within us that is not a part but a state of being, characterized by compassion, curiosity, clarity and calm. When the Self leads, our parts no longer have to fight for control. Over time, they begin to soften, step back and relate to us differently, allowing us to move through life with grounded presence. Yet many of us are unaware that Self-energy is even accessible to us. And even when we are, we may experience our parts in such extreme roles that they overshadow our ability to connect with it. IFS therapy is designed to rebuild that connection to Self-energy, shifting the balance so the Self can lead. As an IFS practitioner, my role is not to "heal" my clients or "fix" their parts, but to help them cultivate their own Self-leadership, because true healing happens when the Self builds trust with our parts.

A Dragon in My Mind

Funnily enough, I discovered IFS in the midst of heartbreak. My partner Sam and I had been in a loving relationship, but when a conflict arose between us that I believed was workable, he shut down instead of working through it. Our conflict stirred up shame he didn't know how to process, and rather than staying engaged, he withdrew. As he grew more unwilling to address what stood between us, I made the painful decision to end the relationship. I realized love wasn't enough if repair wasn't possible.

In the wake of our ending, I initially felt sick with the physical and emotional pain of loss, which then flamed into anger. Extreme anger. During everyday tasks like showering or washing dishes, I found myself embroiled in imaginary fights with Sam—replaying arguments, crafting retorts, saying all the things I wished I had said. The anger took over, waking me up at night, hijacking my daily thoughts and even causing me to lose time as I was temporarily taken over by these dissociative daydreams. I knew I had fallen into the Drama Triangle, but knowing it intellectually didn't help. My usual tools—mindfulness, reframing, grounding techniques—weren't working. I needed something else.

That's when I turned to Jay Earley's *Self-Therapy*, a book based on IFS. His work introduced me to the concept of unblending: the practice of creating enough space between an activated part and the Self so that the Self can stay centered and lead. When a part takes over completely, we become "blended" with it, seeing the world only through its lens. I realized that my Self had been drowned out by the voice of my rage. When I applied unblending, I was stunned. IFS teaches that people perceive their inner parts in different ways—visually, auditorily, viscerally or through an intuitive felt sense. These parts can also take many forms—some humanlike, others more abstract. But when I externalized my anger, it didn't take on a familiar shape resembling me. It became a colossal dragon.

The moment I unblended from it, the dragon stepped outside of me—like a genie released from a bottle, growing from miniature to massive, towering over me in its full intensity. For weeks, this part had been trapped inside me with no way to release its rage. Now, seeing it before me, I grasped the sheer force of what had been burning me from the inside. I wasn't just feeling my anger—I was finally bearing witness to it. I stayed present, tapping into my Self-energy and holding space for this furious part of me. I let the dragon breathe its fire, releasing the rage that had accumulated from the fallout with Sam. Then something unexpected happened. After a few minutes, the dragon calmed. And we began to talk.

This part wasn't just angry about Sam. Its rage had deeper roots—reaching back to other moments of betrayal, loss and unmet needs. This wasn't the first time I had lost someone because they couldn't face their own shame. It had happened in other adult relationships, and even further back, in childhood, with my father's absence. The dragon, fierce and protective, had been trying to shield me from further pain. Its fire was meant to keep people at a distance—to ensure I never let in someone who might hurt me again. But despite the negative impact it was having on me, from Self, I could see its true intention: protection. And so, I listened. I thanked it. And I told it what I hadn't before—that I understood what it was trying to do, but its fire was burning me, too.

We explored how it could still protect me without consuming me. Instead of hijacking me with fury, it could simply tap me on the shoulder to warn me of potential threats. And I would listen. We also decided that rather than living inside me, it would fly outside, circling as a guardian rather than raging within. The moment we made this agreement, the dragon exhaled, its tension easing. Since then, it has become one of my most trusted protectors.

This experience was life-changing. Regaining my sense of Self after unblending from the dragon brought immediate relief. My sleep returned. My presence in daily life resumed. But more than that, it reshaped my entire understanding of healing. I realized that in the past, when I had tried to "work" on my parts, I hadn't been leading with Self. Another part of me had been in control—the part that wanted to *fix* things, to be *done* with an issue, to push forward and override discomfort. I wasn't healing; I was managing. IFS revealed the missing piece: True healing isn't about fixing ourselves. It's about *leading* ourselves. And Self-leadership isn't just a therapeutic technique—it's a way of being, just like all the spiritual practices I had been working with. Spirituality and psychology had finally come together.

Identifying the Shame Triangle

People turn to self-help and personal development because they want something to change. They long for more ease, love, clarity or peace—whether within themselves, in relationships or in their sense of purpose. Over the years, I've picked up countless books, each time carrying the hope that it would provide that elusive *something more*—the spark that would ignite the transformation I was seeking. I see the same longing in my clients. They seek therapy, coaching, courses, psychedelics or spiritual teachings to bridge the gap between where they are and where they want to be. Whether they are struggling with emotional wounds, physical health, relationship dynamics, financial challenges or career shifts, at its core, the search is always about one thing: wanting to feel different than they do now.

Over my years as a therapist and coach, I've had countless conversations with clients about what gets in the way of living their preferred reality instead of being stuck in a problematic one—trapped in a life that feels more like a struggle than a choice. Again and again, the same theme emerges: a relentless inner critic, hammering them with "shoulds" and "shouldn'ts," drowning them in self-doubt, shame and an unshakable sense of unworthiness. They dream of something better—more fulfillment, deeper connection, greater success—but don't believe they deserve it or fear they won't be able to make it happen. Even when they do achieve their goals, the anxiety doesn't end. Instead of allowing themselves to enjoy success, they fear losing it. *What if I mess this up? What if I can't keep it?* The same voices that once told them they weren't good enough now warn them it's only a matter of time before they fail.

While I hesitate to speak in absolutes, nearly every client I've worked with has encountered some version of this inner voice—something that truly stood out to me—even if the particulars vary from person to person. For years, I believed that the Inner Critic was the primary issue. It seemed to be the loudest and most damaging force, keeping people trapped in cycles of shame and self-sabotage. Naturally, I assumed that if we could soften the critical voice—understand it and negotiate with it—healing would follow. But when my clients and I tried to address it directly, something unexpected happened. The problem didn't go away; it *shape-shifted*.

At first, the Inner Critic seemed willing to ease up. My clients would leave sessions hopeful, feeling lighter. But by the next session, the shame was still there, just as strong as before. Or we would focus on addressing self-sabotaging behaviors, only to have our attempted solutions backfire—creating even more distress, avoidance or frustration. No matter how we approached it, the same struggles persisted. It was like a game of whack-a-mole: We'd address one issue, only for it to pop up somewhere else. That's when I realized this wasn't just *one* voice. It wasn't even two. It was three!

At some point, it also hit me that this mess of internal conflict wasn't just a tangle of parts to unravel; it was a *triangle*. A dynamic playing out inside people—an internalized version of Karpman's Drama Triangle that mirrored the external conflicts we experience with others. And once I saw it, I could never unsee it. The Persecutor role manifested as the Inner Critic, relentlessly attacking. The Victim was Shame, absorbing those attacks and collapsing inward. And the Rescuer showed up as the Escapers—a group of parts that, overwhelmed by the battle between the Inner Critic and Shame, each sought relief through strategies like perfectionism, avoidance, numbing, distraction or even more dangerous impulses like self-harm or thrill-seeking.

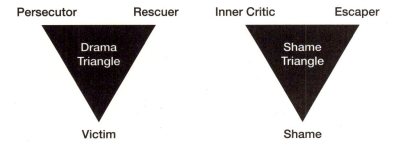

The Inner Critic often initiates the Shame Triangle, launching a barrage of self-judgment—harsh, absolute and unforgiving. But these attacks need somewhere to land, and they find their target in Shame. Shame is the part that absorbs the Inner Critic's words like a sponge, internalizing them as undeniable truth. It doesn't push back or deflect. It accepts the verdict: *I'm not good enough. I always mess things up. I'm too much. I'll never get it right.* Without Shame to internalize these messages, the Inner Critic's attacks would lose their power. But as long as Shame believes them, the cycle remains unbreakable.

The relationship between the Inner Critic and Shame is intense, an endless feedback loop of attack and absorption that necessitates the emergence of a third part: the Escaper, an internal Rescuer who attempts to silence these other voices and escape the resultant discomfort. We can have one or more Escapers, and they can take many forms, each of which uses a different strategy to avoid the tension. One might devote itself to perfectionism, another to overachieving or caretaking, working tirelessly to prove our worth. Or another might take the path of avoidance—scrolling endlessly, binge-watching, overworking, over-drinking or throwing itself into distractions to dull the sting of self-judgment. In more extreme cases, an Escaper might turn aggressive, lashing out at others (what I call the Outer Critic), acting out through risky, high-adrenaline behaviors, or directing its rage inward through self-harm, addiction, or suicidal thoughts. One Escaper part may dominate for a time, until its strategy loses effectiveness or becomes unsustainable. When that happens, another Escaper may step in with a different approach. Often, different contexts evoke different Escaper parts; for example, the Escaper that manages things at work may be entirely different from the one that takes over at home. These Escapers are not just bad habits or character flaws. They are survival strategies—intelligent but misguided attempts to outrun the pain inflicted by the Inner Critic and Shame.

The tragedy of the Shame Triangle is that it traps us in a distorted reality, convincing us that we are broken, unworthy or constantly needing to prove ourselves. It builds walls—between us and others, and between us and our true selves—disconnecting us from our own agency. Instead of making choices based on our values and desires, we become locked in a pattern of reacting to judgment and expectation. The external world might impose social norms, but the Shame Triangle is the *internal* enforcer, ensuring we stay in line. Instead of living for ourselves, we live in reaction—chasing approval, avoiding criticism or shutting down altogether. Under its weight, our lives no longer feel like our own.

Despite the prevalence of the Shame Triangle, I've found that most resources on self-criticism, shame and avoidance treat these three elements as separate issues. There are excellent books on overcoming the Inner Critic, powerful research findings on healing shame and effective strategies for breaking free from escapism. But they rarely connect these three elements as distinct yet *interwoven* parts of a single, self-reinforcing system.

For example, discussions of shame might acknowledge the voice of an Inner Critic, but they frame it as merely a thought process within shame, rather than recognizing it as its own unique force. Similarly, resources on the Inner Critic often neglect to ask a key question: If the Inner Critic is a voice within, then who—or what part of us—is it speaking to? Without identifying the role of Shame, these resources overlook the fact that the Inner Critic's attacks only have power because they have an audience, and together, the Inner Critic and Shame fuel what is commonly referred to as a *shame spiral*. And without addressing Escapers, most resources fail to recognize that addiction, perfectionism, self-sabotage and avoidance aren't just bad habits or an inner disease—they are desperate attempts to navigate the unbearable pressure created by these other two parts.

Additionally, some theories conflate shame with perfectionism or assume it belongs solely to the Inner Child. However, I've found that perfectionism is often fueled by the Escaper, using achievement as a way to escape feelings of unworthiness. That's why, in the Shame Triangle, the Escaper represents a distinct category of parts, each using its own strategy to try to bring relief. And while Shame is often tied to childhood wounds, it isn't *just* about the past. It can form in adulthood and be shaped by culture, relationships and systemic pressures. Similarly, frameworks for escapism, particularly in addiction recovery, may mention Shame but often fail to explore the complex relationships between *all* these parts—how the Inner Critic fuels Shame, how Shame fuels the need to escape, and how all three keep us stuck. Without addressing each of these parts, people can find themselves trapped in cycles of healing work that never seem to reach the root of the issue.

Building on IFS: Similarities and Differences

Some of these ideas may sound familiar to those who have studied IFS, which presents its own internal triangle of Managers, Exiles and Firefighters. At first glance, this model might seem similar to the Shame Triangle, but in practice, I've found key differences. In IFS, Managers work proactively to keep us safe, maintaining control to prevent vulnerability. Exiles carry deep wounds—often childhood pain, shame or trauma—and are typically pushed out of our awareness to protect the internal system. Firefighters react when Exiles' distress surfaces, using impulsive behaviors like addiction, numbing or self-harm to extinguish emotional pain. This creates an internal cycle where Managers suppress Exiles, Firefighters rush in when suppression fails, and the system remains in perpetual conflict.

IFS is one of the most impactful healing models I've encountered, and it continues to shape how I approach inner work. At the same time, through working with clients, I've found that some of its terminology doesn't always resonate in practice. For example, while Firefighters are described as reactive parts, many protector parts I've encountered act both reactively and proactively. This is especially true of Escapers in the Shame Triangle—they might shut down emotionally or zone out by reorganizing the kitchen for the third time or taking an hours-long nap after a shame spiral (reactive), or by micromanaging their schedules and preemptively taking on others' needs to avoid triggering shame in the first place (proactive). Some Escapers are clearly one or the other, while others shift between both strategies depending on what's happening internally and externally.

The Inner Critic, in this model, is a specific type of Manager—one whose strategy is control through judgment, often in an attempt to preempt rejection, failure or shame. While IFS uses the name Exile to describe parts that are pushed out of awareness, I've found that Shame doesn't always function this way. Sometimes Shame is an Exile—buried, suppressed, hidden from view. But other times, it's painfully present, raw and fully blended, dominating our daily experience. And just as not all wounds are hidden, not all protectors are purely defensive—many carry their own burdens. This is why, when working with clients, I often ask, "Is this part holding a wound, trying to protect you, or both?"

IFS offers a broad and flexible approach to parts work, and the Shame Triangle builds on this foundation by focusing on three specific parts—the Inner Critic, Shame and the Escaper—that I've repeatedly found to be at the core of the patterns that keep people stuck. Unless we address all three *together*, we risk falling into endless cycles of self-work that never quite lead to the transformation we long for. This is precisely what *Transforming the Shame Triangle* seeks to address. It provides a focused framework to identify and work with these three parts, allowing us to move beyond coping mechanisms and into true healing. In my experience, we must untangle the Shame Triangle to reclaim our lives. Until we do, we remain locked in the protective strategies of our past, trapped in problem-saturated stories and reactive patterns, rather than stepping fully into the sovereignty of a Self-led life.

The Shame Triangle Journey

The Shame Triangle is adapted from several psychological models, offering a powerful lens through which we can examine the depths of our internal world. It reveals the root of our suffering and provides a pathway toward genuine transformation. In my work, I tend to be skeptical of models that are either too simplistic to capture real-life struggles or so complex that they become impractical. What I strive for instead is a balance: a framework that is nuanced enough to address deep, recurring challenges while remaining accessible and applicable. This journey isn't about quick fixes or psychological shortcuts. It's about efficiently and effectively getting to the core of what holds us back so that we can pursue real, lasting change. That's precisely the work of the Shame Triangle, in my experience.

The Shame Triangle underpins many of the struggles my clients face. Sometimes, it is the main issue. Other times, it is the hidden force preventing deeper healing. Either way, it destabilizes both our inner world and relationships, influencing how we see ourselves and how we move through life. Without addressing it, we find ourselves living on shaky ground—no matter how much self-work we do elsewhere. As in a house without a solid foundation, surface-level changes won't create real stability.

Take a moment to think about an issue you've been struggling with—something that feels stuck or unresolved. Now, ask yourself: Are the voices of the Shame Triangle present in this struggle? Is your Inner Critic attacking you for how you're handling the situation? Is Shame making you feel small, incapable or unworthy? Is the Escaper pulling you toward avoidance, distraction or perfectionism as a way to cope? Sometimes, the parts themselves *are* the issue. Other times, they're amplifying the difficulty—turning a manageable challenge into something overwhelming.

To truly transform the Shame Triangle, we must engage with these parts in an entirely new way. This work involves listening to them with curiosity, offering validation, extending gratitude and love, and setting healthy internal boundaries. Through this process, we can recast them as allies rather than adversaries within our bodies, hearts and minds.

As I shared earlier in the story about my dragon, I discovered that true transformation only happened when Self was the one leading the work; when another part tried to manage the process, it stalled. That realization changed everything for me, and I began to see the same dynamic play out with my clients. When they tried to engage with their Shame Triangle from a perfectionistic part, it would attempt to correct things with affirmations, forcing change through willpower. When they approached the Triangle from a wounded part and met resistance, they would collapse into defeat, reinforcing the belief that they were broken. Even other well-intentioned parts only led to more inner struggle. No matter how we approached the work, if Self wasn't leading, the transformation didn't take hold.

This key is also why many popular approaches—like self-care, self-compassion and self-love—often fall short. These practices, while well-meaning, are easily hijacked by the Shame Triangle when not rooted in Self. Instead of healing, they become more fuel for inner conflict. When the Inner Critic is in charge, self-care turns into a measure of worth—another way to succeed or fail. If you don't meditate, journal or exercise the "right" way, you feel like you're falling short. When self-compassion is filtered through Shame, it feels inaccessible—like something you don't deserve. You may try to force kindness onto a part that simply doesn't believe it. And when self-love is driven by the Escaper, it becomes a way to numb discomfort or distract yourself, rather than truly care for yourself.

The result is that even well-intended self-care practices can reinforce the very struggles they aim to heal. Instead of being sources of love, they become more standards to fail at. This is why being connected to Self is so important. True healing doesn't come from another part trying to control or override the system—it must come from Self. When Self leads, these parts experience something entirely different. They are no longer being attacked, dismissed or pressured to change. They are seen, understood and supported. And that is what allows them to transform. This is where the *Self-Love Triangle* emerges.

The Shift from Shame Triangle to Self-Love Triangle

Once we are centered in Self and leading from it, the Shame Triangle no longer operates as a system of blame, fear and escape. Instead, its parts shift into their highest expressions, creating a new internal dynamic:
- **The Inner Critic becomes the Inner Coach:** a voice that still holds us to healthy standards but does so with encouragement rather than punishment. Instead of attacking, it supports. Instead of tearing down, it builds up.

- **Shame transforms into Raw Experience**: our capacity to fully feel what is. No longer weighed down by the oppressive belief that we are broken or unworthy, we reclaim the ability to experience all emotions as they arise—without resistance, escape or self-judgment.
- **The Escaper evolves into the Inner Nurturer**: no longer numbing or avoiding, but actively turning toward our discomfort with care, comfort and genuine self-support.

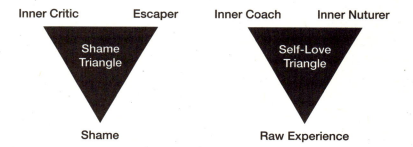

The term Self-Love Triangle is an intentional play on words. Instead of a love triangle's chaotic, conflicted dynamic, this is an integrated inner system of presence, curiosity, acceptance and care. Often, what literature or pop culture refers to as a love triangle is more about possessiveness, obsession and lust than actual love. Here, we are deliberately reimagining the concept—not as a tumultuous romantic scenario, but as an integrated inner system grounded in Self-energy, a triangle of loving relationships between oneself and our different parts. The Self-Love Triangle is an internal state of Self-leadership, where all parts are welcomed into their preferred expression. Where shame and blame once ruled, love now leads.

This transformation is both a destination and a lifelong process. The journey from the Shame Triangle to the Self-Love Triangle is about reclaiming ourselves—not by eliminating or silencing our inner voices, but by helping them evolve. Each part is invited to shed its constricting role and instead embody the love, wisdom and presence that has always been at our core. I'm excited for you to experience this shift firsthand.

About Us: Jess and Dave

Those of you already familiar with me and my work probably already know that my journey to writing this book began long before I put pen to paper or finger to keyboard. I've been talking about transforming the Shame Triangle in interviews, public talks and client sessions for years now. In many ways, I wrote this for you. For those of you who are new to me and my work, it's nice to meet you! Here are a few more basics about me.

I grew up as a third-generation New Yorker in the housing projects of Brooklyn. I was immersed in a neighborhood familiar with violence and a family deeply affected by multiple divorces, multigenerational traumas, substance abuse, mental illness and interpersonal discord. These early experiences posed significant challenges and impacted all areas of my life for many years. However, they also ignited a powerful determination within me. I resolved not only to thrive and be resilient in the face of my childhood hardships but also to contribute to the healing and transformation of others who have been impacted by neglect, abuse, trauma and poverty.

Driven by a desire to understand how to heal the mind, body and heart, as I've shared above, I embarked on a journey of extensive study, exploring everything from spiritual practices to academic theories. I dedicated my life to investigating how we change, evolve and develop; how we can communicate healthily and effectively; how we can heal and become safely embodied in the wake of trauma; how we can unshackle our hearts from survival-based reactivity and defenses; and how we can liberate our minds from bigotry, ignorance and internalized oppression.

Over the past 25 years I have professionally immersed myself in holistic health, psychotherapy, trauma and attachment healing, spiritual counseling, communication and conflict resolution.

Along the way, I became a somatic bodyworker, socially engaged Buddhist, genocide researcher, early childhood development program evaluator, mediator, psychotherapist and author. Having many inner parts has led me to many paths, each one drawing me to new modalities along the way. My experiences and studies culminated in my previous works, including my books *Polysecure* (2020) and *Polywise* (2023), where I explored attachment theory in the context of consensual nonmonogamy and the wisdom of polyamory. These books have resonated with readers worldwide, offering new perspectives on relationships, trauma and personal growth, giving more of a voice to the millions who practice love, sex, relationships and family in ways that differ from societally sanctioned norms.

For this new book, I bring with me not only my personal experiences and professional expertise, but also the insights gained from my previous works, which were written for more specialized audiences within specific subcultures. This time, my aim is broader. This book is for anyone seeking growth, healing and a deeper connection to themselves and others. It represents the next step in my ongoing mission to make these transformative ideas accessible, practical and deeply impactful for a wider audience.

I am also thrilled to be coauthoring with David Cooley again. Dave and I have been in each other's lives since 2002, sharing a meaningful and evolving journey. Over the past two-plus decades, we've navigated the roles of classmates, friends, lovers, husband and wife, co-parents, ex-spouses, family of choice, nesting life partners and coauthors. Our relationship fluidity, marked by a deep commitment to one another and our son, has continually matured as it has ebbed and flowed. We've embraced what works best in our partnership, not forcing what doesn't, truly embodying the essence of not throwing the baby out with the bathwater. Now let's turn to Dave.

> **David here!**

Like Jessica, I come from a richly layered background that has exposed me to different cultural perspectives and realities. Raised in the South, I grew up in social contexts where racial tension, economic hardship and community-level violence were prevalent. Although I belonged to the racial majority in the United States, I grew up in a community where my white identity seemed to make me a frequent target of violence. As a child, this was a deeply disorienting experience—not because I had any conscious expectations about what my race meant, but because the pain and confusion of being targeted felt inexplicable to my young mind. I didn't yet have the language or awareness to understand the broader social forces shaping these dynamics. All I knew was that something felt fundamentally unsafe and unjust, and it left me with a lot of unresolved questions about who I was and why things were the way they were.

Only later, as I sought to understand these early experiences, did I become aware of the larger reality of racial inequality in the United States and the insidious concept of white supremacy that has been at the center of this injustice—the people who perpetrated violence against me were also victims of the larger identity group I belonged to. It was a harsh awakening, one that shattered my illusion of a just and equitable society and left me to question my identity and the weight of my privilege. These experiences left a lasting impression on me, prompting difficult questions about identity, belonging and injustice. Rather than distancing me from these realities, they became a catalyst for my lifelong desire to understand the roots of conflict and to seek meaningful pathways toward healing and repair.

That search led me to the field of restorative justice. As a professional restorative circle facilitator and trainer, I guided people through conflict resolution processes that offered an alternative to the traditional court system. Along the way, I trained in trauma-informed care for crime survivors, cultural and gender sensitivity, nonviolent communication and cultural bridge building. But as my relationship to this work grew, I realized that true conflict transformation required more—it called for a broader, more holistic approach. I began integrating mindfulness-based practices, narrative therapy, somatic work and attachment theory, weaving together a more comprehensive framework for healing and repair.

Yet after years in the nonprofit world, I burned out. I came to a stark realization: Real, lasting healing at the community level wasn't just about policy or intervention—it was about relationships. Without strong, healthy relational foundations, conflict would always find a way to resurface. This shift in perspective led me to reimagine the restorative models I had been working with, adapting them for a more personal, intimate context. I wanted to help individuals, not just communities, develop more sustainable ways of navigating conflict, particularly in their closest relationships. Out of this vision, I created the Restorative Relationship Conversations model, a framework designed to help people repair ruptures, process trauma and cultivate authentic communication and attunement.

Over the years, Jessica and I have discovered a natural synergy in our collaborations, blending our intellectual strengths and shared passion for personal transformation. This dynamic worked beautifully in our last project, *Polywise*, so continuing to work together on this new book felt like an obvious choice. When Jessica first introduced me to the concept of the Shame Triangle, I immediately recognized its relevance: how the Inner Critic, Shame and the Escaper don't just shape individual struggles but also influence the ways people attempt, and often fail, to repair relational conflict. As I wove the Shame Triangle into my restorative relationship work with clients, it became clear that Jessica had uncovered something truly unique—a kind of linchpin or decoder for conflict transformation. Seeing its impact firsthand, I knew without a doubt that I wanted to be part of bringing this work into the world!

From here on out, we'll speak primarily in the "we" voice to reflect our collaboration. When one of us wants to share a

> personal anecdote from our own perspective, we'll switch to first person and make it clear whose voice you're reading.

Our intention for this book is to introduce you to the Shame Triangle framework and guide you in transforming it into the Self-Love Triangle. This work is a unique fusion of our experiences with narrative practice, Internal Family Systems, archetypal work, mindfulness practices, somatic practices, the Drama Triangle, shamanic practices and restorative justice. We have been deeply immersed in all these modalities—personally, professionally or both—for decades. Just as this book is about having multiple internal parts, it is our experience that change, healing and growth require the application and fusion of multiple modalities. Along with sharing these diverse concepts, we provide reflection questions and numerous exercises to help you deepen your understanding.

For true change to occur, this work must be experiential, not just conceptual. Many of the exercises are presented as guided visualizations or inner journeys which may or may not resonate with everyone. People experience their parts differently. While some people have clear internal visuals, others don't picture anything at all. Some people have a nervous system variation called aphantasia that means they struggle to create or access visual imagery, even when trying to imagine something. For them, parts work can feel like navigating without a visual map. But it's entirely possible to do this work without mental images. In fact, Richard Schwartz, the founder of IFS, has aphantasia.

Even within the same person, different parts may come through different channels. One part might show up as a clear image, another as a voice, and another as a physical sensation, shift in emotion or intuitive sense. Some people experience parts as changes in posture, energy or mood. If visualizing doesn't come easily, try tuning into sound, bodily sensation or emotional tone. You can also try accessing the part more directly, such as by speaking as if you are the part or writing from its perspective. Additionally, some parts may feel more like a "who"—a distinct inner presence—while others may feel more like a "what"—a pattern, role, object or symbol that emerges in your awareness. For example, a part might show up not as a personality, but as a color, shape or texture. The key is to experiment and trust your own way in. There's no single correct method, only the one that fits your unique system.

We encourage you to approach these exercises with curiosity and a willingness to try things that may seem different, weird or even silly, as they can help shake up the Shame Triangle and transport you to new, transformative places. Some of these questions and practices may create immediate "aha" moments that drastically alter your inner landscape. Others may result in more subtle shifts, but as in traveling by airplane, a small one-degree shift in course can ultimately lead to an entirely different destination. Similarly, a tiny change in your inner world may not be immediately obvious but will gradually guide you on an entirely new trajectory, far from where your old patterns would have taken you.

With that said, you have full permission to adapt any of our exercises to suit your needs. You can turn a guided visualization or meditation into a journaling exercise, act it out, or use props such as pillows, chairs or action figures to externalize your parts and work with them physically. You can take whatever exercise we initially suggest and dance it, speak it out loud or do whatever suits your process best. The goal is to find what works for you in breaking free from the Shame Triangle and embracing the Self-Love Triangle.

As you engage with these exercises, be mindful of how your inner parts might react. Your Inner Critic might try to convince you you're not doing it "right" or that you're not progressing fast enough. Your Shame part might whisper that you're incapable of making these changes or unworthy of them. And your Escaper part might urge you to avoid these challenges because they threaten the familiar internal status quo. If you notice these reactions, see them as opportunities to practice unblending, connecting with your Self and applying the very techniques this book will guide you through. Remember, transformation isn't an endpoint, it's an ongoing process.

A Note on Shame Versus shame

Throughout this book, you'll notice we use Shame (capital *S*) when referring to it as a part—a distinct aspect of your internal system that carries the weight of shame-based beliefs and stories. This part often exists in multiple forms at different ages, holding onto the problem-saturated narrative that you are unworthy, broken or fundamentally flawed. When we use shame (lowercase *s*), we are referring to the feeling of shame—the emotional response most people are familiar with.

However, we see what is commonly called "the feeling of shame" as something more than just a feeling. It is often a pseudo-emotion, rooted in fear and shaped by an internalized story of deficiency. Unlike emotions such as sadness or anger, which rise and fall naturally, shame tends to linger, distort perception and reinforce itself through an ongoing narrative. Understanding this distinction allows us to work with Shame as a part differently than we would with a feeling. Rather than seeing it as something to overcome or simply endure, we can begin to relate to it as a part—listening to its story, supporting it in unburdening its pain and self-deprecating beliefs, and ultimately helping it transform into something more aligned with our Self.

Book Overview

This book is designed as a step-by-step process for transforming your Shame Triangle. There is an intentional progression to this work, moving from awareness to engagement to transformation.

The goal is that by the end, you aren't just thinking differently about yourself but relating to yourself in a completely new way.

We begin in chapter 1 with the Drama Triangle, a model that helps us recognize patterns of blame, powerlessness and over-responsibility in relationships. Understanding these roles sets the stage for chapter 2, where we turn inward to identify the Shame Triangle—seeing how these parts show up in our lives and what impacts they have, and beginning to create space between ourselves and their patterns. In chapter 3, we explore where these patterns come from—how past experiences, family messages and cultural conditioning shape the ways we relate to ourselves—while also identifying the triggers that activate the Shame Triangle in daily life.

With this awareness in place, we shift toward change. Chapter 4 introduces Self—not as a part, but as the core of who we are. When we are in contact with our Self-energy, we have the ability to truly heal and effectively work with our parts. Chapter 5 builds on this understanding by making Self more tangible. Since Self can feel like an abstract concept, we introduce the Self-centered model, which helps us engage with the mind, heart and body—the three centers where the Shame Triangle takes hold and distorts our experience.

Once we've established this foundation, we begin the work of engaging with the Shame Triangle parts directly. Chapter 6 focuses on beginning a direct dialogue with your Inner Critic, Shame and Escaper to begin reshaping your relationship with them. From there, we apply the Self-centered model to the Shame Triangle, exploring how it plays out in the three core centers of experience. Chapter 7 looks at the Shame Triangle and the body, focusing on nervous system regulation and how different states like fight, flight, freeze and fawn influence your relationship with your Shame Triangle parts. Chapter 8 examines the Shame Triangle and the heart, exploring how our emotional lives have been shaped by the Shame Triangle and how we've built protective barriers around our hearts to avoid vulnerability. Chapter 9 looks at the Shame Triangle and the mind, identifying rigid, adversarial and shame-driven ways of thinking and shifting toward Self-led mindsets that offer more perspective and flexibility.

In the final section, we move beyond personal transformation into a wider perspective. Chapter 10 focuses on inherited burdens—when the Shame Triangle is not just a personal experience, but something passed down through family, culture or collective trauma. You'll learn how to recognize and release burdens that were never yours to carry. Finally, in chapter 11, we bring everything together through a restorative relationship process that allows your Inner Critic, Shame and Escaper to repair with each other and step fully into their new Self-Love Triangle roles.

Δ

Embarking on the journey to explore and dismantle your Shame Triangle is not easy. This work requires bravery and a certain level of safety and stability in your life to support you through the process. If you are currently in an unsafe or abusive environment, you should prioritize your safety first before undertaking this work. However, you do not need to be in a perfect environment or have many resources at your disposal to begin. While this work can be challenging, the benefits of confronting and understanding your Shame Triangle are significant. You can undertake this work by yourself using the guidance provided in this book or with the support of a professional, trusted loved one or peer. Each approach offers unique benefits, and we invite you to seek out the necessary support and structure to help you navigate this liberatory and transformative process.

Liberation is a process of unveiling, where we expose the aspects of the world that no longer fit or serve us. We begin to see the societal norms, expectations and beliefs we've outgrown—the ones that have shaped us but no longer align with who we are. After we become aware of them, we can shed them. We can let go, release and disidentify from the parts of ourselves that hold us back, including not only externally imposed limitations, but also the self-imposed fears and patterns that have kept us bound to old ways of being.

From there, we can begin to rebuild. This is the alchemical part of transformation—where we take what remains and shape it into something new. We don't erase the past or discard our experiences; instead, we turn them into wisdom, strength and a clearer sense of ourselves. This process expands what we believe is possible, opening doors that once felt locked. True transformation isn't just about seeing differently—it's about living differently, with more authenticity and choice. Recognizing and working through the Shame Triangle is both a journey of coming home to ourselves and a process of recreating ourselves. As we transform these parts, we heal and evolve, integrating what we've learned into a fuller version of who we are. Let's begin!

CHAPTER 1
THE DRAMA TRIANGLE

We've all been there—stuck in the same argument, the same frustrating dynamic, the same unresolved tension. No matter how much we hope this time will be different, we find ourselves slipping back into a familiar role, caught in an emotional loop that plays out over and over again. Maybe you feel powerless, unheard or misunderstood. Maybe you're the one pointing out the problem, making sure someone is held accountable. Or maybe you're the fixer, stepping in to smooth things over, to make sure everything stays OK.

Psychiatrist Stephen Karpman mapped out these patterns in what he called the Drama Triangle:

- **The Victim**: "This always happens to me." This part feels powerless, overwhelmed or trapped, convinced there's no way out.
- **The Persecutor**: "This is your fault." This part blames, criticizes or controls, pushing responsibility onto others.
- **The Rescuer**: "I'll fix this for you." This part jumps in to save the day, taking responsibility for others at the expense of our own needs.

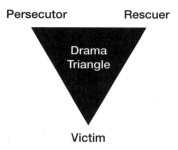

The Drama Triangle is the foundation for understanding how external conflicts become internalized as the Shame Triangle. This model helps us see the reflexive roles we fall into during both conflict and everyday interactions with others, and ultimately with ourselves. No matter which role you find yourself in, the Drama Triangle keeps conflict alive, amplifying emotions and perpetuating ongoing cycles of disconnection, misunderstanding and hurt.

These roles are not set in stone. We often shift between them, sometimes occupying multiple positions simultaneously in different relationships or even switching roles within a single conversation. At first, it's easy to see these patterns in others: an overbearing boss, a guilt-tripping parent, a friend who always plays the martyr. But we play these roles ourselves, too. You might notice you gravitate toward a particular role or find yourself shifting between them depending on the situation. Think back to the last conflict you had, big or small. Maybe you started in the Victim role, feeling unheard and powerless, but then flipped into Persecutor mode—lashing out, pushing back, making sure they knew it was their fault. Or maybe you took on the Rescuer role, bending over backward to keep the peace, trying to make everything better for the other person, but when your efforts weren't appreciated, frustration crept in. Suddenly, instead of a Rescuer, you felt like the Victim—unseen, unappreciated, taken advantage of. And before you knew it, you found yourself in Persecutor mode, blaming the other person for being selfish, ungrateful or unwilling to meet you halfway—convinced that if they weren't so stubborn or dismissive, none of this would be happening.

> *Jessica here!*
>
> For me, an incident involving something as innocuous as bubbles during a family Fourth of July gathering became a memorable illustration of the Drama Triangle. I was about twelve years old that year, and in an effort to avoid the potential injuries associated with fireworks and sparklers, the adults gave us bubbles instead. Initially disappointed, we kids made the best of it. The moment of contention arose when from across the room, I observed my best friend, Kirsten, struggling with her bottle of bubbles because her bubble wand was missing. I watched as she reached into my bottle and took my wand. Thinking it was funny, I expected a playful exchange when I asked with a smile, "Why did you just take my bubble stick?"
>
> Uncharacteristically, Kirsten vehemently snapped back, adamantly denying she took anything from me. Her reaction was shocking and disproportionate, immediately thrusting us into the Drama Triangle. Caught off guard, I replied, "But I just watched you take it," believing that stating the obvious would clear things up. Instead, Kirsten doubled down, calling me a liar and insisting I was making it all up. This accusation hurt and firmly established the dynamic between us, positioning me as the Victim and her as the Persecutor. I couldn't understand why she was lying or why she was calling me a liar. I felt wronged by Kirsten's unwarranted aggression, allegations and petty theft, and my attempts to clarify the situation with the truth of what I saw was only met with her further denial and hostility, which escalated the conflict and worsened our entrenchment in the drama.
>
> Kirsten's defensiveness continued. Her level of obstinance (and what we would now refer to as gaslighting) was something I had never encountered before. At my wits' end with

> the ineffectiveness of my words, I finally slapped her on the side of the head, hoping to knock some sense into her and get my best friend back. Instantly our roles switched. I became the Persecutor, employing physical means to assert my point, while Kirsten became the Victim of my outburst. The moment my hand connected with her head, I knew I had crossed a line. Kirsten ran off crying, and I was left standing there, feeling utterly horrible and at a complete loss to understand what had just happened. Realizing the gravity of my actions, I ran after her to make amends. In doing so, I stepped into the role of the Rescuer, attempting to alleviate the harm I had caused. Tearfully, I offered my heartfelt apologies to Kirsten for hitting her and then I even extended an awkward offer that she could hit me back, in the hope of canceling out what I had done. As Kirsten yelled at me for what had just happened, I remained steadfast in my apologies, letting her air out her anger.
>
> Much like how she and I knew precisely how to push each other's buttons, we equally knew the pathways to each other's laughter. Eventually, by referencing an inside joke familiar only to us, I managed to elicit a smile from her, breaking the ice and opening the way for us to return to our friendship as usual. This gesture put the dynamics of the Drama Triangle on hold, and we were able to have fun for the rest of the party—even creating a new inside joke about stealing bubble sticks—but the underlying pattern was by no means eradicated from our adolescent best friendship.

This incident, seemingly trivial and even ridiculous in the grand scheme of things, serves as a notable example. It illustrates the fluidity with which we can swiftly switch between positions on the Drama Triangle, as well as how quickly such a dynamic can arise and take over, even around something as small as bubbles. In everyday life, many of us also find ourselves unintentionally and without explicit consent caught up in the Drama Triangle with those around us. The tragedy of the Drama Triangle unfolds when, in our interactions with those important to us, we resort to communication laced with blame, criticism, contempt or defensiveness. These kinds of responses position us against one another, often over matters that either held no antagonism in the first place or could have been resolved through kinder and more constructive dialogue. It's easy to look at Jessica's story and dismiss it as just childhood drama, but the truth is, these same patterns play out in our adult lives—in our relationships, at work, online and even on the world stage.

Social media is rife with Drama Triangle dynamics. People post experiences of being wronged, casting themselves as Victims. In turn, others rally to their side, offering support and criticizing the alleged wrongdoer—stepping into the Rescuer role. Meanwhile, some commenters attack either the original poster or their supporters, taking on the role of Persecutors. This dynamic rarely fosters the empathy or help people truly need—it simply perpetuates more drama.

Of course, people are sometimes truly harmed, victimized and in need of assistance. But engaging in the Drama Triangle doesn't actually help. It locks people into rigid roles that fuel blame, outrage, polarization and helplessness rather than resolution. We see this play out in politics, news and international relations. Entire nations frame themselves as Victims, justifying their retaliation as self-defense. Others take on the Rescuer role, intervening under the guise of aid, though their true motivations may align more with self-interest than actual support. Even in the face of real oppression and injustice, these roles keep conflict in place, preventing the meaningful solutions needed for lasting change.

From the personal to the political, at the root of the Drama Triangle is a form of victim consciousness—a state of mind where people see themselves as powerless, perpetually at the mercy of external forces. This mentality is defined by a sense of helplessness, where a person believes their happiness, circumstances and suffering are dictated by others or by situations beyond their control. Entrenched in victim consciousness, people adopt a narrative of external blame and unaccountability, believing they are being wronged, that they have no real choices or that their emotions are solely the fault of someone else. This mindset removes personal agency, placing responsibility entirely on external factors. In essence, it traps people in a problem-saturated story, where they feel like life is happening to them rather than through or with them.

Operating from victim consciousness changes how we see the world. It compels us to perceive external forces—other people, systems, circumstances—as the ultimate orchestrators of our experiences. Within the Drama Triangle, each role is either an expression of victimhood or an attempt to escape it.

- **The Victim** embodies this mindset most clearly, feeling targeted, wronged and powerless to change their situation.
- **The Persecutor** takes an aggressive stance, preemptively striking out to avoid becoming the victim themselves (perhaps thinking *If it weren't for the victim, I wouldn't have to be so harsh*). But there is also the **righteous Victim**—a person who, having felt victimized, believes they now have the right to punish, attack or control others as a form of justice. This belief fuels cycles of retaliation, where one person's victimization becomes the justification for their persecution of someone else.
- **The Rescuer** swoops in to save others, either to avoid facing their own sense of helplessness or to keep themselves from being cast as the Victim or Persecutor in the story.

This is how the Drama Triangle self-perpetuates. Each role, in its own way, is a response to the same core discomfort of being powerless. Whether we're seeking to control, mend or escape, we're still operating from the belief that we are at the mercy of something outside of ourselves.

Why So Much Drama?

Karpman frequently describes the Drama Triangle as an expression of the "games people play," and notes that these are not necessarily enjoyable games of the playful variety, but rather the kind where there are no true winners. Despite each participant's earnest attempts to win, be right or at least be justified in their position on the triangle, such interactions inevitably culminate in scenarios where all parties are worse off. Karpman's reference to these situations as "games" implies that there's an inherent part of us that revels in the act of playing, even when the outcomes seem futile. We think there's some truth to this idea, which raises the question: If the Drama Triangle is so damn dysfunctional and a relational dead end, rife with stress and trauma, why do we persist in engaging with it?

The answers are multifaceted. For one, there's the adrenaline rush we get from conflict, which, despite its discomfort, can also be exhilarating and habit forming. Conflict can become addictive due to the cascade of neurochemicals it sets off, which elevate our heart rate, heighten our senses, boost our energy and sharpen our focus. This natural rush can create a sense of heightened vitality, making the experience of conflict both stressful and invigorating, and it can also serve as a temporary escape from the mundanity or stressors of daily life, providing a momentary feeling of empowerment or euphoria. This feeling can create a cycle where people seek out conflict or high-stress situations as a means to experience these effects again, chasing the adrenaline-fueled high. The brain's reward system reinforces this cycle, seeking out conflict and its intensity in a potentially addictive pursuit that intertwines physiological excitement with psychological gratification, albeit short-lived.

Additionally, those with a history of abuse, neglect or trauma may become primed for a heightened threat response. In such states, we may not consciously seek conflict, yet our brains swiftly propel us toward it as a defensive mechanism aimed at ensuring our safety. This response is based in the logic of our more primitive brain structures which, especially under stress or trauma, operate on the principle that it's better to erroneously perceive a threat than to overlook one. Consequently, we find ourselves in a state of hypervigilance, which significantly increases our susceptibility to falling into the archetypal roles of the Drama Triangle.

Another factor driving our inclination toward the Drama Triangle is the simple fact that, for many, it's all we've ever known. From an early age, this model of interaction was ingrained in us as the standard way people relate to one another. If conflict, blame or scapegoating were the norm in our childhood homes, we learned to accept these roles, not because they were healthy, but because they were familiar. Beyond the home, these dynamics often extended into the environments where we grew up: bullying in school hallways, clique culture, toxic academic competitiveness or even harsh punitive discipline, all reinforcing an atmosphere of power struggles and emotional manipulation. Over time, these patterns have seeped into broader social arenas, where politicians lean on "us versus them" narratives, media thrives on drama and oppressive power structures further normalize these roles.

When these dynamics are so pervasive, it's easy to mistake them for the natural order of things, to assume they're just how people interact, rather than seeing them as patterns that perpetuate harm. Our engagement in the Drama Triangle, then, isn't always a conscious choice. More often, it's a reflection of the social and familial environments we've inherited. In spaces shaped by unequal power dynamics and learned patterns of conflict, the Drama Triangle can become an unconscious default, pulling us into the roles of Victim, Persecutor and Rescuer without us even realizing it.

As we look further into how our social structures shape our affinity for the Drama Triangle, consider the broader trend of disciplinary justice systems worldwide. Across the globe, approaches to crime and conflict vary widely, from harsh punitive models to more rehabilitative ones. In nations that embrace a "tough on crime" philosophy—marked by strict sentencing and high incarceration rates—the Persecutor-Victim dynamic is reinforced at a systemic level. Even without realizing it, on a personal level, we absorb these values and language, framing relational conflict in moralistic, zero-sum terms with clear winners and losers. When someone wrongs us, we instinctively brand them as a "wrongdoer" who deserves punishment, mirroring the very mindset that turns everyday conflicts into high-stakes drama.

This punitive mentality seeps into nearly every aspect of our lives—how we parent, how we handle stress, how we drive, how we navigate disagreements with partners, friends or colleagues. The idea of "being in trouble" also looms large, shaping how we respond to mistakes. Whether at home, school or work, or in public, missteps often come with penalties—being grounded, losing privileges, getting fired, being fined or even facing legal consequences. Over time, we internalize the belief that loss of privileges or rights is the natural consequence of personal failure, rarely stopping to question whether punishment actually leads to learning and repair.

From a young age, many of us are also taught the importance of being "good" and an "upstanding citizen," reinforcing the idea that breaking rules isn't just about consequences—it tarnishes our very identity. This link between wrongdoing and moral failure fosters a deep sense of shame in the face of conflict. The real issue isn't just that mistakes come with consequences; it's that we are conditioned to believe those consequences define us. In this environment, we learn to stay on constant alert, fearing not only punishment but the damage to our self-image that comes with it.

Conversely, consider people who grow up in environments where authority figures—such as parents, teachers or law enforcement—consistently view them through a lens of suspicion or disapproval and interpret their behavior in the worst possible light. For example, when neurodivergent students act out in class, their teachers might punish them harshly rather than trying to understand them. In another instance, teenagers of color are often stereotyped as troublemakers by school administrators and disproportionately targeted by law enforcement. And some children grow up in strict homes with parents who overreact to minor mistakes and respond with harsh, punitive consequences.

Over time, the people subjected to these harsh judgments may internalize them, concluding that there is no point in trying to be "good." Some then embrace roles like bully, outcast or rebel as a form of self-protection, shielding themselves from further rejection in a world they believe will condemn them anyway. This creates a self-reinforcing cycle: The more a person is labeled as "bad" and subjected to punishment, the more likely they are to keep acting out, not as a reflection of who they truly are, but as a response to how they have been seen and treated. Instead of addressing the root causes, these negative labels become entrenched, making change feel impossible and leaving the deeper wounds unhealed.

Another compelling factor drawing us toward the Drama Triangle is its tangible payoffs. We take on these roles not only because they provide familiar patterns of interaction, but also because they can meet certain emotional or psychological needs in the absence of more fulfilling alternatives. Negative attention can be preferable to none at all, so when our core relational needs for power, worth, attention and care go unmet, we may then pursue what is more readily available to us. Each role on the Drama Triangle offers the temporary fulfillment of certain needs, even if that fulfillment is short-lived and comes at a high cost.

Table 1. Drama Triangle role payoffs and costs

Role	Payoff	Costs to Self	Costs to Others
Victim	The role of the Victim can be irresistible because it allows people to avoid taking responsibility for their actions and circumstances, and to instead shift the blame to others. It can elicit sympathy and support and can reinforce a sense of being cared for and connected.	Remaining in the Victim role fosters feelings of powerlessness, low self-esteem and limited personal growth. Relying on external sympathy creates dependence and often strains relationships, making it difficult to break free from helplessness.	The Victim's persistent helplessness can place strain on relationships, especially when others feel pressured to rescue, fix or accommodate. It can provoke frustration or resentment and reinforce dynamics where mutual responsibility and growth are obstructed.
Persecutor	The Persecutor role can be tempting because it offers a sense of power, moral superiority and control over others. By blaming or criticizing the Victim, the Persecutor asserts dominance, which can be compelling for people seeking authority or struggling with helplessness and shame.	This role often leads to emotional isolation; recurring cycles of anger, guilt and shame; and damaged relationships. The Persecutor's need to control or criticize masks deeper vulnerabilities, making it difficult to experience intimacy, trust or personal healing.	The Persecutor's aggression or judgment fosters fear, defensiveness and low self-esteem in others. Victims often feel diminished, while Rescuers may become overextended trying to mediate or pacify. These dynamics erode psychological safety and mutual respect.
Rescuer	This role is appealing because it provides a sense of value and purpose through helping or saving others. It feels good to be needed. The Rescuer receives appreciation and gratitude, strengthening their self-image as a caretaker or savior.	Constant rescuing often results in burnout and resentment—especially when efforts go unappreciated—and can lead to neglect of the Rescuer's own needs and growth.	The Rescuer's actions also prevent the Victim from developing personal agency and autonomy, reinforcing the belief that they are powerless, perpetuating dependency and hindering personal accountability and growth. It can also provoke irritation or resistance from the Persecutor, escalating the triangle rather than resolving it.

Additionally, adulting is hard. As modern life increasingly moves us away from communal support systems, taking full responsibility for our lives becomes daunting as it requires us to navigate complex emotional, financial and social terrains without the guidance of elders, the solidarity of peers or the support of equitable institutional structures. For this reason, the opportunity to evade responsibility or defer it onto others adds to the allure of the Drama Triangle, making it seem attractive for managing the complexities of adult life.

Another reason the Drama Triangle can be so compelling arguably stems from an intrinsic human trait: our ability for storytelling. Researchers suggest that, at our core, it is not our thinking brain that makes us uniquely human, but our proclivity for storytelling. Our brains are wired to perceive and interpret the world through stories. Using narrative structures like myths, legends, fairy tales, rhymes, songs and oral histories, we organize information, shape reality, frame memories, forge connections and construct identities that help us understand and navigate the complexities of life. This human penchant for storytelling is seen as a universal trait crossing all cultures and all eras, which suggests that it is a central feature of human cognition and social bonding. The concept of *Homo narrans* ("storytelling human") was first proposed by German ethnologist and folklore expert Kurt Ranke (1967, translated to English in 1981) as a more apt descriptor than *Homo sapiens* ("wise human") because it emphasizes storytelling's unique significance in human evolution and the way it distinguishes us from other species, even more so than our intelligence and logical reasoning.

The earliest traces of human storytelling, discovered in caves over 30,000 years old, hint at the key role of firelit gatherings in our ancestral narrative traditions. These ancient gatherings around the fire served to pass down important knowledge, cultural values and traditions from one generation to the next, as people embedded lessons of survival, morality and the human experience within captivating narratives. Today, much of our storytelling still revolves around the same essential themes. Roles like victim, villain and hero—nearly identical to those Karpman named in the Drama Triangle—appear across everything from ancient scripture to modern entertainment (our current version of gathering around the fire). In fact, when you look at the highest-grossing films of all time, nearly all of them are expressions of the Drama Triangle dynamic: stories built around good versus evil, oppression and resistance, tragic love or the rise of a hero. These stories, full of complex characters and moral dilemmas, not only hold our attention (and money) but also reflect our strong attraction to tales that embody the Drama Triangle dynamic through adversity, heroism and redemption.

This affinity for drama through entertainment mirrors more than just our love of a good story—it reflects the very way we understand and navigate life itself. Joseph Campbell's concept of the monomyth, or "one myth," posits that all mythic narratives are variations on a singular grand story: the hero's journey ([1949] 2008). This journey is characterized by overcoming obstacles, often including villains, and undergoing transformation. Campbell's theory recognizes a universal pattern underpinning the narrative elements of great myths across different cultures and eras, and it highlights our enduring connection to stories that echo the Drama Triangle. Campbell's work suggests that the hero's journey resonates deeply because it speaks to our intrinsic desire for transformation—yet we often remain stuck in cycles of conflict without reaching resolution. The tragedy of the Drama Triangle lies in our struggle to break free from its grip; rather than evolving beyond its roles, we find ourselves repeating them, leaving the potential for personal and collective growth unrealized.

Finally, while the Drama Triangle is deeply embedded in our cultural narratives and storytelling traditions, it also has a biological basis in our stress response system. When we engage in Drama Triangle dynamics, we're often operating from a state of nervous system dysregulation, which pushes us into fight, flight, freeze or fawn responses rather than balanced, intentional reactions. We'll explore the body's stress responses in more depth in chapter 7, but it's important to briefly touch on them here because they help explain why the Drama Triangle feels so instinctive and why it can be so hard to break free from it. Our fight, flight, freeze and fawn responses are built-in survival mechanisms designed to protect us from danger. When activated, they bypass conscious thought and dictate how we respond to conflict and stress. These responses don't just show up in life-or-death situations—they also appear in our emotional and relational experiences, including when we are on the Drama Triangle. Here's how that typically looks for each response:

- **Fight** (Persecutor): Responding to perceived threats with aggression, blame or control in an attempt to regain power.
- **Flight** (Rescuer or Victim): Avoiding conflict by physically or emotionally escaping, distracting oneself with busyness, or focusing on fixing others instead of facing personal struggles.
- **Freeze** (Victim): Becoming paralyzed in the face of conflict, feeling helpless, numb or unable to take action.
- **Fawn** (Rescuer or Victim): Attempting to appease or over-accommodate others to avoid conflict, maintain safety or seek approval.

These physiological responses explain why Drama Triangle dynamics feel so immediate and difficult to escape—they're not just psychological patterns or familiar relational roles, but instinctual survival reactions. When our nervous system perceives a threat, even if it's emotional rather than physical, it releases stress hormones like adrenaline and cortisol. As mentioned, this flood of chemicals sharpens our focus and increases our energy, creating a natural high that can become addictive. Some people unintentionally return to drama again and again because, despite its destructiveness, it provides a familiar sense of arousal, intensity or purpose.

Additionally, stress puts the brain in survival mode, causing us to think in black-and-white terms and see others more quickly as adversaries. This narrowed perspective makes it harder to access the higher brain functions responsible for empathy, perspective-taking and problem-solving. When we are dysregulated, we are more likely to fall into Drama Triangle roles, and once we're there, the dynamics themselves cause further stress, creating a reinforcing loop. However, not everyone engaged in Drama Triangle dynamics is constantly in acute stress. For many, these roles become habitual—low-level stress states we live in without even realizing it. But whether the stress is chronic or flares up in moments of acute conflict, the impact is the same and our nervous system keeps us bound in the cycle. Understanding this connection between stress and the Drama Triangle helps explain why these patterns can feel so hard to break, even when we know they're not serving us.

Who Starts the Triangle?

Any of the three roles can kick off the Drama Triangle. All it takes is someone directing blame at another—assigning someone else responsibility for their own feelings, the circumstances or a larger issue. Once blame is introduced, the dynamic unfolds, pulling others into the cycle.

If the Persecutor casts the first stone, they point an accusatory finger at the Victim, asserting power or control through criticism, judgment or aggression. This assertion allows them to maintain their position of superiority, believing they are justified in their actions. In response, the Victim feels hurt, insulted or powerless, convinced they have no control over what's happening. Seeing their distress, the Rescuer—either summoned by the Victim or stepping in uninvited—tries to alleviate the Victim's suffering, though often without addressing the actual underlying issue.

Victims can also set the Drama Triangle in motion. Instead of waiting for a Persecutor, they may project the role of the Persecutor onto others, their circumstances or the world at large. Viewing life through a lens of opposition, they perceive adversaries—real or imagined—everywhere, turning outward to assign blame. This perception shields them from taking responsibility for their own challenges while reinforcing a belief that they are at the mercy of forces beyond their control. Additionally, Victims often seek Rescuers to save them, preferring dependency over autonomy. However, this dynamic becomes self-defeating, as Victims may crave help while simultaneously dismissing or resisting it, believing their situation is uniquely unsolvable.

Finally, the Rescuer can spark the Drama Triangle through well-intentioned but unsolicited, forced or counterproductive attempts at help. Often driven by a need to be needed or by a desire to avoid confronting their own issues, Rescuers jump in to solve problems for others. However, their interventions often disempower the Victim, reinforcing helplessness and dependency rather than fostering true support. In some cases, their efforts may even cause resentment; those they are trying to help may feel patronized, undermined or controlled. Ironically, the Rescuer may be seen as the real Persecutor, offering "help" that isn't actually helpful. Additionally, by prioritizing others' problems over their own, Rescuers often neglect their own needs and boundaries, leading to burnout, frustration and unappreciated efforts. When their help is refused or fails to produce the desired outcome, the Rescuer can feel victimized themselves, blaming others for taking advantage of them or not appreciating their sacrifices.

Ultimately, no matter where the triangle begins, the roles are fluid and interchangeable. Each one can morph into the others, keeping the cycle alive, entangling people in maladaptive roles that repeat over and over again. Table 2 provides an overview of the Drama Triangle roles and common statements or beliefs associated with them.

Table 2. Drama Triangle roles and beliefs

Role	Also known as	Description	Statements
Persecutor	Villain, Bully, Aggressor, Blamer	People in the Persecutor role often seek to assert dominance or control over others, using criticism and blame to maintain power. They respond with anger or criticism when challenged. They easily feel insulted or offended. Both the Victim and the Rescuer tend to see the Persecutor as the cause of the Victim's plight.	"It's your fault!" "You brought this on yourself!" "I'm just telling it like it is—if you can't handle it, that's your problem." "You're to blame for messing up and making me angry." "What's wrong with you?"
Victim	Target, Oppressed, Scapegoat, Underdog, Injured Party	People in the Victim role experience a sense of powerlessness, oppression and helplessness. They often believe they have no agency to solve their problems and that they must endure their suffering. They feel persecuted and picked on by the world at large and focus on being abandoned, rejected and insulted. They take things personally.	"Poor me!" "How could they?" "Nobody understands me." "Oh, you think you've got it bad? You don't even know what I'm dealing with!" (competitive victimhood) "I can't do anything right." "Nothing I do ever makes a difference."
Rescuer	Hero, Martyr, Enabler, Caretaker	The Rescuer strives to alleviate the Victim's suffering, frequently by offering unsolicited help or support. Although this support can seem altruistic, it discourages the Victim's self-sufficiency and fosters dependency. Rescuers seek to alleviate pain without addressing the actual underlying issues. They are usually averse to being perceived as a Persecutor. They may deny their own needs or avoid supportive equal relationships.	"I need to be needed." "I can't ask for help." "I'm the only one who can fix this." "I have to do it all by myself." "If I don't do it, it won't happen."

Getting Off the Drama Triangle

The rest of this book is focused on the way we internalize the Drama Triangle as the Shame Triangle, and how we can transform the Shame Triangle within ourselves. But before we move on, we want to at least offer a few ideas to help you get off the Drama Triangle as it plays out in your relationships with others. Here are three steps to get off the Drama Triangle: self-awareness, self-regulation and self-accountability. Another, pithier way to remember these steps: "catch it, calm it and change it."

Self-Awareness (Catch It)

The first step to getting off the Drama Triangle is recognizing that you're on it. It is only by seeing the Victim, Persecutor and Rescuer roles within our own behaviors and interactions that we can begin to dismantle the drama that binds us. Awareness creates choice. We can't change what we can't see, and once we recognize that we've fallen into the Drama Triangle, we gain the ability to consciously interrupt and shift our habitual responses.

To strengthen this awareness, it's important to understand the personal cues that signal you've entered the Drama Triangle. These may show up as emotional reactions, physical sensations, recurring thought patterns or certain behaviors that emerge when you assume these roles. Becoming attuned to these signals allows you to catch yourself in the moment, marking your entry onto the Drama Triangle and giving you the opportunity to step off before the cycle continues.

To cultivate this awareness, here are some points and questions to consider:

Awareness of Drama Triangle Archetypes

- Think about the media you consume (movies, TV shows, books). How are the Persecutor, Victim and Rescuer archetypes typically portrayed? Do you notice any

patterns or stereotypes in these representations? Which do you resonate with or resist?
- Think about politicians or celebrities who embody these archetypes. Can you identify public figures who consistently play one of these roles in their public persona or interactions? How do these portrayals influence public perception and discourse? How have they impacted you?
- Consider also how these three archetypes might manifest in different cultural contexts. Have you seen variations in how these roles are perceived or expressed in different societies or subcultures? Reflect on the myths or stories from your own culture or religion, or even the stories you've heard about family members growing up. How do these narratives reinforce or challenge the Drama Triangle roles? What impact do these stories have on your beliefs and behaviors?

Awareness of Your Emotional and Physical Cues

- Think of a time you were on the Drama Triangle. What feelings and emotions did you experience? Did you experience anger, frustration, helplessness or the impulse to jump in and save others?
- What are the physical signs that you are on the Drama Triangle? What happened in your body? Physically, did you feel tension, a racing heart or a sense of heaviness?

Awareness of Your Thoughts and Stories

- Reflect on the quality of your mind and the kinds of stories and thoughts you have when you're on the Drama Triangle.
- What is the quality of your mind when you are on the Drama Triangle?

- What kinds of thoughts do you have? Are they accusatory, self-deprecating or overly concerned with another's welfare at the expense of your own?
- What types of problem-saturated stories do you start to tell yourself or others when you are stuck in a Drama Triangle part?

Awareness of Your Role

- **Persecutor:** First, tune in to how this role shows up in your interactions. In what situations or relationships do you notice yourself overtly or covertly dominating, bullying or judging others?
- **Victim:** Notice how this role appears in your interactions. In what situations or relationships do you feel powerless, seek sympathy or rely on others instead of taking initiative?
- **Rescuer:** How does this role show up in your interactions? In what situations or relationships do you find yourself offering unsolicited advice or taking on others' responsibilities?
- **Role Preference:** What role do you find yourself in most often? Why do you prefer this role or feel more comfortable with it than with the others? Are there any roles that repel you or that you have an aversion to taking on? If so, why?

As you reflect on each role, ask yourself:
- What are you trying to achieve by assuming this role—validation, control, value or an escape from your own issues?
- What payoff do you get from being in this role?
- What are the costs?

Triggers and the Drama Triangle

By identifying specific situations, words or behaviors that propel you into these roles, you can anticipate and manage your reactions more effectively.
- What external or internal stimuli trigger you into entering the Drama Triangle?
- What patterns do you notice that tend to precede slipping into one of these roles?

Impact on Others

Consider the effects of your behavior on the dynamics of the situation and on the other individuals involved.
- How do your actions impact others within the triangle?
- How about people around you who might not be in the Drama Triangle with you?

Self-Regulation (Calm It)

Once we recognize that we are on the Drama Triangle, the next essential step is self-regulation. As discussed earlier, being caught in these dynamics is often a sign of nervous system dysregulation. When our body perceives conflict or emotional tension as a threat, it instinctively shifts us into fight, flight, freeze or fawn mode, pushing us into the reactive roles of Persecutor, Rescuer or Victim. Self-regulation is what allows us to step back, regain control over our emotions and respond with intention rather than reactivity. In chapter 7, we provide more specific self-regulation practices, so for now, we'll simply emphasize its importance.

The key is to pause as soon as you recognize you're on the Drama Triangle. This brief moment of awareness gives you the chance to calm your nervous system and bring yourself back into regulation. Creating a small space between stimulus and response allows you to step out of automatic reactions and make a conscious choice. Techniques such as deep breathing, grounding exercises, mindful body awareness, or movement-based practices like shaking, stretching or dancing can help release built-up energy and bring your system back into balance. These practices enable you to assess the situation with a clearer perspective and choose a response that aligns with your values. The more we practice self-regulation, the more accessible it becomes. Over time, this skill helps us navigate difficult situations without defaulting to the Drama Triangle's dysfunctional patterns.

Reflection Questions

- Think of a recent situation where you found yourself on the Drama Triangle, feeling either heightened or shut down. What set off this state of dysregulation? Describe what it was like and how you reacted. How would you have preferred to respond instead?
- What are some methods you already use to self-regulate when you feel stressed, angry, anxious, afraid or dysregulated? How effective do you find these strategies in helping you return to a state of calm and clarity?
- Can you recall a time when you successfully managed to pause and calm yourself before responding in a stressful situation? What did you do to achieve this pause, and how did it change the outcome of the situation?
- Considering your current methods of self-regulation, what new techniques or practices could you incorporate to enhance your ability to manage emotional and physiological responses? How might improving your self-regulation impact your roles within the Drama Triangle?

Self-Accountability (Change It)

The final step in getting off the Drama Triangle is practicing self-accountability—taking ownership of your actions and choices and their impact, rather than blaming others or external circumstances. While we can't control what others do, we do have control over how we respond. One person choosing accountability can shift an entire dynamic. Don't underestimate your ability to be an agent of change. Taking responsibility doesn't mean blaming yourself—it means recognizing your role in the interaction, owning your part and then considering what you can do differently moving forward. This shift from reaction to intentional action is what ultimately allows us to step off the Drama Triangle and engage in relationships with greater clarity, integrity and empowerment.

Own Your Participation

To help you identify your participation in the Drama Triangle, we offer a question: How did I *cause, contribute* to or *condone* the situation? This question moves from the most to least active forms of participation, helping you gain clarity and be accountable for your actions. In any Drama Triangle situation, you can ask:
- **Cause:** How did you cause, kick off or otherwise initiate this situation?
- **Contribute:** Maybe you did not start the situation, but how did you actively contribute to, influence, escalate or participate in it?
- **Condone:** How did your lack of action passively condone the situation or allow it to occur? How did you stay passive through silence, inaction or avoidance?

What You Can Do Differently Moving Forward

The next step in self-accountability and fostering change is to explore what you can do differently next time. This process involves setting clear intentions for how you want to handle similar situations in the future. By consciously guiding your actions and responses, you increase the likelihood of staying off the Drama Triangle—or at least stepping off it more quickly once you recognize you've fallen into it. Changing these patterns comes down to three key behavioral shifts: asserting without persecuting, embracing vulnerability without succumbing to victimhood, and supporting without overstepping.

Persecutor → Assertive Advocate

Persecutors start to shift when they move from control to clear, grounded assertiveness. Instead of using power to punish or dominate, we can use assertiveness to speak up without shutting others down. It's how we set boundaries, name harm and advocate for ourselves—while still respecting the humanity of the other person. When we're anchored in this kind of clarity, we don't have to rely on blame or shame to get our point across.

Assertiveness also helps us recognize the difference between calling out and calling in. Sometimes, it's necessary to call someone out—to publicly name harmful behavior, especially when there's urgency or safety at stake. But even then, we can focus on the impact of the behavior instead of attacking the person. Other times, we may choose to call someone in—inviting them into a real conversation, one that's honest, direct and actually goes somewhere. When people aren't being shamed or attacked, they're far more likely to stay open, take in feedback and consider change.

If you recognize yourself in this role, ask:
- How can I assert my wants, needs and boundaries while still respecting those of others?
- How can I challenge what feels wrong in a way that invites change rather than defensiveness?
- How can I express my concerns constructively rather than reactively?
- What boundaries do I need to establish to avoid slipping into controlling behaviors?

Victim → Conscious Participant

Victims transform when they recognize their ability to respond—to make choices, take action, and influence their experience, even in the face of unfair circumstances. Being a Conscious Participant means stepping out of passive helplessness and into active engagement with life. It doesn't mean ignoring hardship or pretending everything is within your control, but it does mean acknowledging what is. Even when you can't change a situation, you can change how you relate to it.

Also, stepping out of the Victim role doesn't mean denying your emotions or avoiding difficult conversations. You can acknowledge harm and express hurt without being passive or powerless. Speaking up about your pain, setting boundaries and advocating for your needs are acts of strength—not victimhood.

If you find yourself feeling like a Victim, consider:
- What choices do I have in this situation, no matter how small?
- How can I take an active role in creating change in my life?
- What is within my control, even if it's just how I see this situation?
- How can I express hurt or harm in a way that invites repair rather than reinforcing blame or powerlessness?

Rescuer → Attuned Supporter

Rescuers transform when they balance caring with respect for others' autonomy. Instead of stepping in to solve problems for others, a healthier approach is to offer support while empowering others to find their own solutions. This strategy fosters growth, independence and healthier relationships, rather than reinforcing dependency. A key shift here is getting consent before offering help and asking what kind of support is genuinely helpful, rather than assuming. Attuned Supporters develop greater awareness of what is truly needed, ensuring their help is constructive rather than enabling.

If you recognize yourself in this role, reflect:

- How can I offer support without taking over?
- How can I encourage others to take responsibility for their own challenges?
- Am I stepping in because they truly need help, or because I feel uncomfortable watching them struggle?
- How can I be more attuned to what is helpful and supportive rather than assuming?

These role transformations encourage a shift away from dissatisfying patterns of interaction toward more balanced, respectful and supportive relationships. By being assertive without being punitive, vulnerable without being passive and supportive without being disempowering, you can create more functional and supportive dynamics.

Of course, we cannot control how others choose to show up in relationship to us. People who are invested in perpetuating Drama Triangles may repeatedly try to cast us into familiar roles. When this occurs, we can request that they relate to us differently and we can set boundaries around problematic ways of relating. You can share the impact that being on the Drama Triangle has on you and the relationship, you can suggest creating agreements to avoid these roles, you can provide tips for healthier interactions, and you can point to resources to help them learn. Professional support can also help reinforce new patterns. However, sometimes people are unwilling or unable to shift away from the Drama Triangle. In such cases, you may need to create more distance from the relationship to protect your well-being. Ultimately, our self-responsibility lies in how we are accountable for our part, choose how we show up to interactions and decide how close we can be to others who refuse to relate in respectful ways.

∆

The Drama Triangle reflects the fundamental human desire for validation, power and connection. We lash out when we feel unheard. We shrink when we feel powerless. We step in when we feel needed. But true connection exists beyond these two-dimensional roles. When we stop seeing ourselves and others through the rigid lens of Victim, Persecutor and Rescuer, we begin to interact from a place of self-awareness rather than habit, self-regulation rather than reactivity and self-accountability rather than blame. This shift allows us to navigate relationships with greater ease, creating interactions that feel more safe, genuine and fulfilling. These shifts are more than just concepts—they are game changers. As you experiment with these ideas in your interactions, we hope you experience how relationship altering they can be.

Now that we have this understanding of the Drama Triangle, we can turn our attention inward to the Shame Triangle.

CHAPTER 2
GETTING TO KNOW YOUR SHAME TRIANGLE

In the last chapter, we explored the Drama Triangle: the constellation of archetypal roles that keep us trapped in interpersonal conflict. Now, we want to understand how these roles become internalized, forming the Shame Triangle: three parts that together create an internal drama that turns our inner world into a battleground, pits us against ourselves and keeps us reactive rather than responsive to life. For your life to truly be your own, it's essential to recognize and understand these three parts rather than be ruled by them. Conceptually understanding the Shame Triangle is one thing, but getting to know how it operates inside of you is another. This chapter is our first step in getting to know these parts. To do this, we'll use narrative therapy–inspired questions designed to help you externalize the parts, giving you more perspective so they feel less fused with your identity.

So far, we've described the Shame Triangle as consisting of one Inner Critic, one Shame part, and one or more Escapers. However, many people can have more than one Shame Triangle, each shaped by different experiences and influencing distinct areas of their life. For example, you might have an Inner Critic tied to your career that operates like a drill sergeant, berating you to work harder, be smarter and never show weakness. Meanwhile, a different Inner Critic might pipe up in your relationships, acting more like a harsh gatekeeper, warning you that if you express too much, need too much or reveal your flaws, others will leave. Each of these critics is potentially connected to different Shame and Escaper parts. Your triangle parts may also be different ages. For example, a child Shame part may hold the pain of being ashamed for wetting the bed at a sleepover. A teenage part may feel humiliated for being publicly dropped by their crush. Meanwhile, an adult Shame part may carry the weight of losing a job and struggling to find work. Each of these Shame parts holds a different wound from different stages of life. The same is true for Inner Critic and Escaper parts: They can be different ages and reflect different life experiences.

If you find that you have multiple Shame Triangles operating in different areas of your life, that's completely normal. These patterns form in response to different influences and recognizing them helps you see how they function separately and where they might overlap. The goal is not to collapse them into a single pattern, but to understand the unique ways they show up so you can begin to work with them more effectively. As we get into these questions, if you feel ready to explore all three parts in one sitting, great. But if you'd rather take your time and focus on one part at a time, that's just as valuable. Move through this process at a pace that feels right for you. What matters most is that you engage with it.

The Inner Critic

The Inner Critic can come in many forms and flavors, varying in its intensity from mildly annoying to outright vicious. In its less severe form, the voice of our inner persecutor can nag and nitpick, functioning like a persistent shadow casting doubts and whispering critiques of our decisions, actions, and even unspoken thoughts and feelings. This intermittent voice can question us with "what if" scenarios concerning the minutiae of our lives, nudging us into a maze of second-guessing, guilt and regret over both our actions and our inactions. Much like a squirrel in a frenzied dash to collect and stash away nuts for the winter, our Inner Critic accumulates our slightest missteps, storing them away for endless rumination. In this guise, the Inner Critic may subtly blend into our sense of self, leading us to mistakenly believe it's an inherent attribute or intrinsic part of our personality rather than recognizing it as a distinct, and often harmful, internal voice. In its milder forms, the Inner Critic can operate almost invisibly, like a low-grade hum in the background—always there, even if we're not consciously aware of it. It often disguises itself as everyday habits we consider "responsible" or "practical," like the constant need to stay busy or productive. We rarely slow down enough to realize it's actually the Critic's fear of not measuring up. It polices us and pre-emptively criticizes us before others can, trying to hide any evidence of our flaws so that no one else sees them. Over time, these patterns feel so normal that we stop questioning them. What seems quiet isn't always quiet—it's just so familiar we've stopped noticing it. Because this voice has been with us for so long, we assume it's just the way things are, rather than something we can challenge or change.

As the volume of our Inner Critic intensifies, it can become a prophet of doom, conjuring scenarios of danger with every "what if" and enveloping us in a haze of indecision or outright panic. Using catastrophic thinking, our Inner Critic amplifies our fears and activates our nervous system, transforming manageable situations into overwhelming crises in our minds. By telling us that our every potential move is a prelude to disaster, the Inner Critic locks us in a state of perpetual fear, stifling our ability to move forward with confidence and clarity. In this version, the Inner Critic normalizes its chronic fretting as a prudent approach, where we begin to mistake its litany of disastrous *what might happen*s and *if only I had*s as the voice of reason. When we believe this voice, it undercuts our ability to trust in our own skills, experiences, insights and decision-making. Cloaked in an illusion of pragmatism, the Inner Critic embeds itself as a necessary part of our being, convincing us that it's providing needed risk assessment rather than corrosive self-doubt.

Conversely, instead of having a rousing effect, the Inner Critic can also show up as a minimizer, downplaying our feelings and experiences with dismissive remarks like *It's not that big of a deal, Get over it, Stop overreacting* or *Don't be a [fill in the blank]*. This version attempts to shut down our emotional responses, operating under the misguided notion that any display of feelings or vulnerability signifies weakness and should be avoided at all costs. In doing so, it denies us the opportunity to process and navigate through our emotions, stunts our growth and mutes our genuine self-expression. By erecting a facade of toughness or indifference, this version of the Inner Critic equates strength with the conquering of emotions, a belief that impedes our emotional resilience and alienates us from the fullness of our emotional lives.

In its most severe incarnation, the Inner Critic evolves beyond annoyance, worry or suppression into an inner abuser, wielding words like weapons and adopting a posture of aggression and ruthless criticism over anything and everything, both real and imagined. Its tone is one of outright hostility, contempt and belittlement through corrosive insults, slashing personal attacks and grandiose generalizations about our worthlessness and guaranteed future failure. Basically, we're disgusting, we're garbage, we should have never been born. It's cruel and even sadistic. The typical Inner Critic is like those rumble strips on the highway that are meant to alert you with a mild vibration when you've drifted out of your lane. Just as those grooved strips are designed to jolt you back into your proper course, the Inner Critic's purpose is ostensibly to steer you back when you stray from what it deems the "right path." It tries to keep us in our lane in life so we don't get criticized by others, acting as a self-appointed protector against external judgment and rejection. However, at the Inner Critic's most intense level, the rumble strip is lined with sharp nails that will burst your tires when you drive over them. This extreme Inner Critic doesn't offer a gentle nudge. Instead, it completely disables and derails you, viciously shredding you apart and immobilizing you. Rather than serving as a course-correcting alert, it becomes an implement of destruction.

> **David here!**
>
> I can vividly remember the origin of one of my most active and crippling Inner Critic voices. It took root in my sophomore year of high school, in the fluorescent-lit classroom of Mr. Calloway, my English teacher. He believed in rigor, in discipline, in the ruthless sharpening of thought until all excess sentimentality was stripped away. I, on the other hand, wrote with feeling, following the currents of emotion rather than the rigid scaffolding of formal argumentation. The difference between us was a constant point of contention. Ostensibly, his critiques were preparing me for the expectations of university professors—and, by extension, the real world—but I experienced them as a relentless dismantling of something deeply personal.
>
> Day after day, I sat in his class with a sinking feeling in my stomach, dreading the moment my papers would be returned. I poured myself into them, writing with raw emotion, letting my thoughts spill onto the page in a way that felt natural and unfiltered. But when Mr. Calloway handed them back, I cringed at the sight of his red ink slashing through my words like a crime scene. "Too sentimental. Lacks discipline. No clear argument." To drive the point home, he would often address the class with remarks like, "Some of you still write as if this is a personal journal. That won't cut it out there in the real world."
>
> The sting of his disapproval burrowed deep in me. I had always been a sensitive kid, feeling my way through language

rather than structuring it like a blueprint. But Mr. Calloway's critiques went well beyond my grammar or organization; I internalized them like an indictment of the way my mind worked, the way I expressed myself. Each time I turned in an assignment, I braced myself for his disappointment, and little by little, I began to edit myself before my pen even touched the page. I learned to write how he wanted—detached, structured, intellectual—trading my natural voice for the safety of approval.

Over the years, I perfected the art of sounding competent and controlled, yet as an adult I've often been told that my writing feels too disembodied, dry and overly intellectual. The irony is painful. That severance—the one that began in Mr. Calloway's classroom—has followed me ever since. I internalized his voice as my own, an Inner Critic that flares up whenever I dare to write from the heart. Jessica has seen this firsthand in our work together. When she asks me to write stories, to tap into the same warmth and emotion that come so easily when I speak, I struggle. The Inner Critic hijacks the process, steering me toward analytical detachment instead. Yet outside of "serious" writing, I have no trouble expressing feeling, whether in a heartfelt card to a friend or in conversation, where stories flow effortlessly. It's only when writing takes on an official, public form that the critic takes over, demanding that I strip away what makes my voice my own.

That's the legacy of Mr. Calloway. It illustrates how an Inner Critic doesn't just appear out of nowhere—it's shaped by the voices we absorb, the expectations we try to meet and the parts of ourselves we learn to hide to belong. Over time, what starts as external critique becomes an internal law, dictating not just how we express ourselves, but who we believe we are allowed to be.

Mapping the Effects of Your Inner Critic

Here, we provide a set of narrative practice questions designed to help you flesh out the impact the Inner Critic has on you and gain a more comprehensive understanding of how this internal voice operates. You can go through these questions more than once for different versions of your Inner Critic.

Origins

- When did the Inner Critic first make its appearance in your life?
- What specific factors or events contributed to its emergence?

Frequency

- Is it a constant presence, or does it appear only occasionally?
- What situations seem to activate it or amplify its voice?
- Can you identify patterns in how the Critic's voice might be stronger or weaker about different aspects of your life (e.g., work, relationships, self-image)?

How It Manifests

- Reflect on moments when your Inner Critic has been particularly active.
- Can you identify specific situations where it tends to emerge, whether as a nagging presence, a prophet of doom or an outright abuser?
- If you could create an archetypal character of your Inner Critic, what would that be? What would you name it?

The Inner Critic's Go-To Phrases

- What phrases or messages does your Inner Critic repeat most often?
- What are its core beliefs or headline messages?
- Does it sound like anyone from your life or past?

The Inner Critic's Strategies

- What strategies, techniques, deceits and tricks does your Inner Critic use to maintain its influence over you?
- How does your Inner Critic speak to you to impose its authority and maintain control over your thoughts and actions?
- Does it convince you with "what if" scenarios, catastrophic thinking or forecasts of danger and disaster?
- How does the Inner Critic influence your ability to handle everyday challenges? Can you recall a time when it distorted your perception of a manageable situation?
- Does your Inner Critic convince you it's just being practical? If so, reflect on occasions where you mistook the Inner Critic's voice for a pragmatic risk assessment. Did this perspective hinder your trust in your own skills and decision-making?

Emotional Impact

- How does the Inner Critic make its presence known emotionally?
- What other feelings or thoughts does it provoke?
- Consider times when your Inner Critic has led you into catastrophic thinking. How has this forecasting of disaster affected your ability to process experiences and handle everyday challenges?

Navigating Emotional Suppression

- Think about times when your Inner Critic has minimized your feelings or experiences. How did it do this?
- How has this dismissal of your emotions affected your ability to process and express them?

Self-Perception

- How has the Inner Critic affected your self-perception?
- What problem-saturated stories has it made you believe about yourself?
- How do you think it has influenced how you believe others see you?
- When the Inner Critic is in control, what happens to your dreams for the future?

Behavioral Impact

- How has the Inner Critic influenced your actions and decisions, particularly in moments of stress or self-doubt?
- What does the Inner Critic push you to do?
- What does it prevent you from doing?
- Can you identify instances where it led you to act out of character?
- How does the Inner Critic keep you from stepping outside of your usual patterns or taking healthy risks that you know would serve you?

Relationship Effects

- How has the Inner Critic impacted your relationships with others?
- What problem-saturated stories does it tell about others?
- Does it create doubt, mistrust or distance in relationships?

Taking It In and Taking a Stand

Before you move on, take a moment to sit with all of your reflections. It's probably a lot. And honestly, we hope you don't like it. That discomfort matters. Feeling the full weight of the Inner Critic's impact is an essential step in beginning to separate yourself from it. In narrative therapy, this is called taking a stand against the problem—the process of naming what is no longer sustainable for us and recognizing that just because something has been present for a long time doesn't mean we have to accept it as permanent. This isn't about making the Inner Critic the bad guy or waging war against it. It's about deciding that its unchecked influence is not something you want for yourself anymore. It's also about taking a stand for yourself—for your dignity, your voice, your right to be treated with respect inside your own mind. It's about acknowledging that while this part may have served a function at some point, the way it operates now is harmful—and you have the right to question and change that.

Moments of Power over the Inner Critic

One way to support this shift is to recognize the moments where you have already had influence over the Inner Critic—the times when you resisted its strategies, pushed back against its authority or weren't as deeply affected by it. Acknowledging these moments helps remind us that we are not always powerless against the Inner Critic, even if it sometimes seems that way.

- Have there been moments in your life where the Inner Critic did not take over? If so, what was different about those situations?
- Have there been times when you disagreed with the Inner Critic or pushed back against its voice? If so, what allowed you to do that?
- What about that situation prevented the Inner Critic from fully taking control?

- Are there areas of your life where the Inner Critic has had little influence? If so, why do you think that is?

Externalizing the Inner Critic

These questions are designed to help you continue to engage with the Inner Critic as a separate entity, inviting you to playfully alter its distance, shape, size, genre and voice. By interacting with your Shame Triangle parts in this way, you can gain new perspectives, view these parts from different angles and reclaim more of your own power in relation to them.

Characterization

- If your Inner Critic had a physical form, what would it look like? What color, shape and size is it?
- If your Inner Critic were a character or object, who or what would it be?
- Imagine, describe, draw or artistically represent its appearance, size or any distinguishing features.

Size and Distance

- Imagine placing your Inner Critic in the farthest corner of the room. How does that feel?
- Now, picture it outside the room entirely. What changes do you notice in yourself?
- If your Inner Critic appears larger than you, try shrinking it down. How does this affect its influence?

Genre Shift

- If your Inner Critic were in a movie, what genre would it be—a horror villain, a dramatic antagonist or a comedic foil?

- Try "changing the channel" on your Inner Critic. How would it appear in a different genre? For example, how might it transform from a horror movie villain to a character in a sitcom or period piece, from a psychological suspense to an anime or nature documentary?
- Visualize your Inner Critic as a cartoon character. How does this change your perception of it?

Voice Alteration

- Play with changing the pitch, tone and accent of your Inner Critic and notice if and how that feels different.

Shame

If our Inner Critic is the part that internally beats us up, then Shame is the part that hears these criticisms and believes them. As our Inner Critic berates us in the second person with rhetorical questions and accusations—such as *How could you?, Why did you?, You should have, What's wrong with you?*—Shame internalizes these messages, replying in the first person with a resigned acceptance: *You're right: I am broken, not enough, too much, unlovable, crazy, unworthy or deficient.* While Shame may not wish these self-assessments to be true, it becomes thoroughly persuaded by the Inner Critic, adopting the Critic's view as an absolute truth about itself, thus cementing a deeply ingrained belief in our fundamental inadequacy.

This foundational belief system is key to understanding Shame and our approach to working with it as a part. Remember, we are defining Shame as the part that believes and embodies the conviction that we are inherently flawed, broken, unlovable or unworthy. Shame is often the most sensitive and innocent part of us. It holds our rawest need for love and belonging—but it also carries the belief that we're either not enough or too much in all the wrong ways and if we're truly seen, we'll be humiliated beyond repair. To Shame, exposure is more than risky or uncomfortable—it can feel like death or a kind of psychic annihilation. That's why it hides, shrinks and collapses so quickly. This view renders us powerless to effect change, leaving us to conceal ourselves as the only recourse to hide our perceived defectiveness. This sense of powerlessness actively undermines our belief that we can have agency in our lives: The more we view our circumstances as predetermined reflections of our flawed selves, the more convinced we are that positive change is out of our reach.

Like all parts, Shame operates on multiple levels and to varying degrees of intensity. Its spectrum ranges from mild, fleeting moments of self-doubt to intense, engulfing waves of self-hate. As such, it affects our sense of worth and belonging in diverse ways. On one end of the spectrum, we might experience Shame as a subtle discomfort, a nagging sense of not fitting in, not meeting expectations or wishing we wore different clothes today. On the other, it can feel like an overwhelming force, convincing us we are utterly disconnected from those around us and that our life is not worth living.

When our Shame is stuck in the story of its own inadequacy, it becomes a deflated part that feels awful and powerless about who it is. Shame then instinctively seeks to minimize its presence, to fold inward, make itself small, become invisible or dissolve entirely in an effort to circumvent disapproval or abandonment. Although the impulse to retract and hide makes sense in light of these defeatist beliefs, it frequently leads to dissatisfaction and disconnection, as it prevents authentic self-expression and genuine relationships. Shame also hampers self-exploration and creativity, as the fear of judgment or discovery of our perceived flaws can inhibit personal and artistic expression. It is a double-edged sword that, while aiming to safeguard against social exclusion, ends up limiting our ability to engage fully and meaningfully with the world.

When blended with Shame, we often experience a form of deflated narcissism, a state where we focus intensely on ourselves, but through a lens of negativity and deficiency rather than grandiosity. Unlike traditional narcissism, which inflates a person's sense of worth to unrealistic heights, deflated narcissism sinks them into a mire of perceived failure and unworthiness. When Shame takes over, we start interpreting everything—what people say, how they act, even neutral events—through a lens of being fundamentally too much or not enough. Instead of seeing situations as complex or multifaceted, we take them as proof of our inadequacy, bad luck or unworthiness. Every interaction feels like further evidence that we are the problem. This reinforces a cycle of self-focus and self-criticism devoid of self-empathy or ability to see the perspective of others.

When we are entrenched in our Shame parts or trapped in a state of deflated narcissism, our relationships with others inevitably suffer. When our Self is eclipsed by Shame, we deflect the love that people offer to us and hold back the love we could give. In this state, it becomes nearly impossible to truly attune to others. In our work with people in intimate relationships, one person's Shame frequently underpins persistent conflict patterns by compromising their capacity to offer empathy or take accountability and their ability to process their partner's feedback and needs without resorting to a shame-driven defense mechanism. A partner's constructive feedback, reasonable requests or legitimate expressions of need are misinterpreted as criticisms, leading to defensive reactions that divert attention from addressing the core issues at hand.

Shame convinces us of our inability to bring about positive relational change or fulfill our partner's requests, pushing the relationship into a deadlock of unmet needs and unresolved conflicts. The challenges of our Shame not being able to receive constructive feedback and the overwhelming sense of hopelessness to address such feedback coalesce into an Escaper defense mechanism—fight, flight, freeze or fawn—that stifles open dialogue and understanding. This scenario can propel us into adopting a victim role within the Drama Triangle with our partner where we may view ourselves as misunderstood, wronged and powerless. This victim stance intensifies the drama, as it invites a counterresponse from our partner, potentially casting them unwittingly into the role of Persecutor or Rescuer. Despite how obvious Shame can sometimes be, we don't always recognize the ways it quietly shapes our thoughts, behaviors and reactions. At times, it's clear and overwhelming. Other times, it operates beneath the surface—hidden in plain sight, even when we don't consciously feel ashamed.

> ***Jessica here!***
>
> That's how I used to experience shame. When I first encountered Brené Brown's research on shame, I recognized its significance but mistakenly believed I was largely unaffected by it. I wasn't someone who visibly collapsed under self-doubt, so I assumed it didn't apply to me. But that wasn't true at all. My misconception wasn't because I didn't feel shame, but because other parts of me kept it skillfully hidden. My Inner Critic prevented me from acknowledging any Shame parts, viewing any admission of shame as shameful in and of itself, while my Escapers diverted my attention through emotional avoidance, overachieving, spiritual seeking and being overly involved in others' lives. As a result, Shame was mostly exiled from my everyday awareness—even those closest to me couldn't see it. Yet it showed up in both subtle and overt ways that I simply didn't recognize as Shame—zoning out with excessive screen time, emotional eating, avoiding things I truly wanted, feeling panic before public speaking or sinking into crushing episodes of existential nihilism where I questioned the very purpose of my life. Looking back, I can see how extensively the Shame Triangle was operating beneath the surface, limiting my life in ways I didn't fully understand. Often, we don't realize the hold Shame has on us until we finally learn what to look for.

For some people, the presence of the Shame Triangle is much more obvious, like a virus infecting the mind. Psychologist and mindfulness teacher Tara Brach (2003) describes shame as a "trance of unworthiness," highlighting its mind-altering power to overtake our psychological landscape. Being caught in a Shame Triangle spiral can feel like a bad acid trip—distorting your perception of yourself and your surroundings so intensely that it magnifies flaws, erases virtues and drives you deeper into self-loathing. In these disorienting spirals, the Inner Critic seizes control, pulling you even further from self-compassion. When Shame becomes this severe, addressing it can't be a peripheral or casual effort. It must be the central focus of your healing, so you can regain stability and a clear sense of direction in your life.

A final note on getting to know your Shame. People often distinguish between *toxic shame* and what's sometimes called *healthy shame*—the idea being that one crushes our sense of self, while the other helps guide us back to our values and relationships. Often, what's labeled as *toxic* is treated as something to avoid or eliminate entirely, as if all shame is corrosive by nature. But we see it a little differently. We don't view the feeling of shame or the parts of us that carry it as toxic. What creates a toxic internal environment is the story or belief that we are fundamentally flawed, unworthy or broken. Shame can attach itself to that story, often working in tandem with the Inner Critic.

But shame as a feeling—before it fuses with that story—is not inherently harmful. Emotions like remorse, embarrassment, regret or guilt can be important messengers. They show us when we've strayed from our values, when we've been hurt or have hurt someone else, and they remind us of our need for connection. When we allow these emotions to surface without attaching them to a story of personal failure, they tend to move through naturally. We can feel regret without believing we are broken. We can feel embarrassment without deciding we are unlovable. Shame becomes harmful when it calcifies into a fixed identity—when it convinces us that we *are* the flaw. That's what keeps us from seeing the truth: that we are always more than our worst moments.

Mapping the Effects of Shame

This set of narrative questions is designed to help you explore the impact of your Shame parts and gain clarity about how they shape your thoughts, emotions and behavior. You can start with the Shame part that's connected to the Inner Critic you just worked with, and you can also use these questions for any of your other Shame parts. Some prompts—especially those in the Origins section—may be helpful to consider across multiple Shame parts, allowing you to notice common threads or distinct differences in how Shame has developed and shows up in your system.

Origins

- When do you first remember experiencing feelings of shame?
- What specific factors or events contributed to the emergence of your Shame parts?
- Can you pinpoint moments in early life or relationships that seemed to lay the groundwork for these feelings and parts?

Frequency

- Is Shame a constant presence in your life, or does it appear occasionally?
- What situations or environments seem to activate it or amplify its intensity?
- Are there predictable patterns—perhaps around certain people, tasks, personal desires, goals or certain social spaces—that give Shame more power?

How Shame Manifests

- Think of moments when Shame has been particularly intense.
- Can you identify specific situations where it tends to surface in forms such as feeling judged, making mistakes or perceiving that you've "failed"?
- If Shame were an archetypal figure or character, how would you describe it? Does it have a particular tone, demeanor or personality?
- What are the recurring messages Shame tells you about yourself or the world? Do you notice certain phrases or headline messages that Shame repeats?
- Does it sound similar to anyone from your past, or echo certain cultural or familial beliefs?

Shame's Strategies

- How does Shame maintain its hold over you? What does it do to keep itself in place?
- Can you recall a time when Shame distorted your perception of a manageable situation and made it feel overwhelming?
- Have there been moments when you mistook Shame's narrative for a realistic assessment? How did that undermine your trust in yourself?
- How did you come to recognize that it wasn't actually true or that it was only part of the story?

Emotional Impact

- How does Shame show up in your body and emotions? What does it feel like when it takes hold? Does it make you want to hide, withdraw, lash out or shut down?
- What emotions tend to ride alongside shame—fear, sadness, anger or helplessness?

- Can you recall a time when Shame made you feel exposed, judged or inadequate? How did that experience shape how you saw yourself or how safe you felt with others?
- How does Shame affect your ability to be emotionally present with yourself or with people you care about?
- When you're feeling shame, what becomes harder to access—compassion, curiosity or connection?

Self-Perception

- What has Shame led you to believe about who you are at your core? Are there problem-saturated stories you've adopted about your worth or capabilities because of Shame?
- How do you think Shame influences how you believe others see you?
- When Shame is running the show, what happens to your dreams for the future or your sense of what's possible?

Behavioral Impact

- How has Shame affected your actions and decisions, especially in moments of stress, risk-taking or self-doubt?
- What does Shame push you to do—for example, withdraw, over-apologize or hide your accomplishments?
- What does it prevent you from doing, such as pursuing dreams, going certain places, voicing your truth or taking healthy risks?
- Can you identify instances where Shame caused you to act out of character or stifled your creativity?

Relationship Effects

- How has Shame affected your relationships with others (friends, family, romantic partners, coworkers)? Are there

certain stories it uses to interpret other people's actions or words as judgments on your worth?
- Recall a situation where Shame made receiving constructive feedback feel like a personal attack. How did you react, and what effect did that have on the conversation or relationship?
- Think of a time when your negative self-perception, fueled by Shame, distorted how you interpreted someone else's intentions or comments. How did that shape the dynamic between you?

Distinguishing Between Toxic Narratives and Valuable Emotions

- Identify an emotion commonly associated with Shame, such as embarrassment, remorse or guilt. Can you separate the genuine emotion—"I feel sad or hurt about this situation"—from the toxic narrative—"I'm inherently bad/unworthy"?
- What do these shame-based storylines look like for you?
- In contrast, what does it feel like to simply acknowledge a mistake or a moment of embarrassment without leaping to a conclusion about your worth?

Taking It In and Taking a Stand

Before moving on, pause to notice how it feels to see the full scope of Shame's influence. That discomfort—if you feel it—is important. Taking a stand doesn't mean trying to stamp out every trace of Shame; it means recognizing that these limiting stories about who you are or what you deserve can be challenged and revised. You have the right to question the story, rewrite Shame's scripts, and take a stand for the feelings, needs and parts of you that the story is trying to cover up. This is a moment to take a position and choose what you want to carry forward, and what you're ready to lay down.

And if you didn't feel discomfort? That's OK. Not everyone has a strong emotional response. Sometimes, we've gotten so used to Shame's voice that it blends into the background, or other parts of us step in to keep the intensity at bay. Taking a stand doesn't require a dramatic reaction. It can come from a simple recognition and the decision to stop letting old narratives define you.

Moments of Power over Shame

Use these prompts to continue externalizing Shame—seeing it as separate from who you are.
- Are there times in your life when Shame did not take over, even in situations that might typically trigger it? What was different about those situations?
- Can you recall moments when you recognized Shame's narrative for what it was and responded differently? What helped you do that?
- Are there areas of life—certain relationships, passions or hobbies—where Shame's grip feels weaker? Why do you think that is?

Externalizing Shame

Just as in the Inner Critic exercise above, here you will externalize and play with your Shame part to create more distance, perspective and agency in relation to it.

Characterization

- If your Shame had a physical form, what would it look like? What color, shape and size is it?
- If your Shame were a character or object, who or what would it be?
- Imagine, describe, draw or artistically represent its appearance, size or any distinguishing features.

Size and Distance

- Imagine placing your Shame in the farthest corner of the room. How does that feel?
- Now, picture it outside the room entirely. What changes do you notice in yourself?
- If your Shame appears larger than you, try shrinking it down or vice versa. How does this affect its influence?

Genre Shift

- If your Shame were in a movie, what genre would it be—a drama, a mystery, a coming-of-age story, a romantic comedy or a melancholic indie film?
- Try "changing the channel" on your Shame. How would it appear in a different genre?
- Visualize your Shame as an animated character. How does this change your perception of it?

Voice Alteration

- What does your Shame's voice sound like?
- Play with changing the pitch, tone and accent of your Shame and notice if and how that feels different.

Escapers

The Inner Critic is the voice that broadcasts harsh and judgmental stories about us, and Shame is the part that absorbs those stories as truth. Our Escaper—or multiple Escapers—is eager to mute the cacophony. It seeks to silence those distressing voices and exit the scene to seek refuge elsewhere. However, in its attempts to avoid the intense and painful dynamic between the Inner Critic and Shame, the Escaper merely changes the form of our suffering instead of eradicating it.

Escaper parts can take many forms, and we may have multiple Escapers at any given time. Each one is a distinct protector that emerges in its own way, with its own strategy to evade the pain of hearing self-judgment and feeling shame. One prevalent Escaper part leans into overfunctioning, often through overachieving, perfectionism, excessive caregiving, overprocessing of emotions or meticulous planning. These behaviors are propelled by the hope of securing status, approval, recognition and affection, all in an effort to counteract feelings of unworthiness. Beneath them all is the belief that our worth isn't inherent—it has to be earned. Consequently, if you have an overfunctioning Escaper part, you may get trapped in a cycle of tirelessly laboring to "earn" your value. Yet no matter how much you achieve or how much you give, it's never quite enough. All this overactivity may look like it's about proving yourself to others, but it's just as much about proving something to your Inner Critic—hoping that if you do enough, it will finally back off, quiet down or give you a break.

In stark contrast to the hustle of overfunctioning, another Escaper works through underfunctioning: retreating by zoning out, numbing, spacing out, dissociating or losing ourselves. We might procrastinate, overindulge in distractions like binge-watching, scroll endlessly through social media, overeat, anesthetize ourselves with substances, lose ourselves in video games or get lost in fantasy worlds through books and movies. These activities offer a refuge from reality, creating a buffer that dulls the edges of our experiences and emotions and using numbness as a shield against the pain and complexity of our inner and outer worlds.

We want to be clear that these behaviors, when practiced intentionally and in moderation, can be perfectly healthy ways to relax and decompress. Casual phone scrolling, enjoying a glass of wine to unwind, watching a show to take a break from a stressful day, enjoying a treat or playing video games are all valid forms of leisure. However, the concern arises when they become tools of evasion. Instead of using these activities to recharge, the underfunctioning Escaper uses them to avoid any more input from our Inner Critic and Shame. They morph into strategies to sidestep our emotions, relationships and responsibilities, creating a perpetual pause and distancing us from the very essence of living and experiencing life in its everyday fullness.

However, not all underfunctioning Escapers are trying to feel nothing—sometimes they're just trying to feel something else. Rather than face the raw pain of Shame, we might escape into emotional states that seem more tolerable or socially acceptable, like anxiety, panic, irritability, anger or depression. In other cases, we might escape into overfunctioning positivity—becoming overly hopeful, enthusiastic, cheerful or idealistic as a way to sidestep harder emotions. These emotions may seem productive or even admirable on the surface, but they can function just like any other Escaper strategy: as a way to keep Shame at a distance. Even when they're intense, these emotional states can feel more familiar or "allowed" than shame, which often feels too exposing or unbearable to touch. So instead of numbing out, our Escaper may shift to express these other feelings, creating the illusion of emotional expression while still avoiding the core wound. We might not realize we're escaping Shame at all because these other emotions feel so consuming or socially reinforced, but in many cases, they're a smoke screen that shows up to protect us from the deeper feelings underneath.

Another variant of the Escaper emerges as an aggressor, acting out either externally toward others or internally toward ourselves. In its outward expression, this aggressive Escaper transforms into an Outer Critic, projecting its internal criticisms outward instead of grappling with our own Inner Critic and Shame. This outward projection can range from silent judgments and an air of disapproval or arrogance, to more overtly confrontational behaviors, where the Escaper turns into the Persecutor, aggressively critiquing, attacking and belittling others as a form of self-evasion. Some Escapers seek to escape through intensity—engaging in risky, high-adrenaline or thrill-seeking behaviors such as reckless driving, substance use, dangerous sexual encounters or infidelity. These strategies often create a temporary high or numbing effect that distracts from inner pain, but ultimately deepen cycles of disconnection and shame. While these high-intensity, thrill-seeking Escapers seek relief through external risks, others direct the same intense energy inward.

When this aggression is directed inward, the Escaper can either amplify its underfunctioning tendencies to dangerous levels, where overindulgence spirals into addictive behaviors, or become more overtly self-destructive. This might include acute self-harm such as cutting, engaging in dangerous or reckless activities, or contemplating or attempting suicide. This internal aggression from the Escaper represents a desperate and often understandable attempt to escape from internal pain and turmoil, but it often intensifies the very suffering it seeks to avoid. Self-harming Escapers are seen as taboo and can evoke strong reactions from others, often propelling them onto the Drama Triangle. People might jump into the Rescuer role to offer support, step into the Persecutor role and harshly criticize you as "selfish," or take on the Victim stance, reacting with disbelief that you could even consider doing something like that to them.

A self-harming Escaper is a more extreme variation and requires immediate support. We view self-harming Escapers as parts that need help distinguishing between the pain they want to end and the person themselves: This Escaper mistakenly believes the entire person must end to find relief. However, when someone whose Self is blended with an Escaper in this extreme form is guided to unblend, access their Self separately and offer genuine understanding and care to their Escaper part, new alternative options emerge.

While the self-harming Escaper shows us the most extreme form of this part's attempts to escape pain, Escapers don't always start in moments of deep suffering. Often, they begin in the smallest of moments, in childhood, in tiny pivots away from discomfort. These early escapes can seem harmless until they solidify into patterns that shape the way we relate to uncomfortable feelings for the rest of our lives.

> ***Jessica here!***
>
> My first memory of implementing an escape strategy is from when I was around five years old. My grandmother had my cousin and me over for a sleepover. Usually, we girls slept in the same bed, but this time Grandma wanted us to sleep in separate rooms, which meant only one of us would have the comfort of Grandma singing lullabies while tucking us in. It also meant one of us would sleep in the room everyone in the family thought was haunted or, at the very least, cold and creepy. Grandma, being all about fairness, decided my cousin and I should do a best of two out of three coin tosses to determine who would get Grandma to sing them to sleep, while the other would have to fall asleep alone in the haunted room.
>
> I lost the coin toss and as my cousin celebrated, my face and posture revealed how scared and disappointed I was—and Grandma immediately scolded me: "Jessica, don't be a sore loser!" At five years old I couldn't yet anticipate how upset I'd be if I lost, and now I also felt ashamed for feeling bad. Instinctively, I came up with a way out. I insisted I wasn't upset about losing, but completely unrelated to the coin toss, I had just remembered that, when I was two, my great-grandfather died, and he had given me a penny the last time I saw him. The penny from the coin toss reminded me of him, and I said I was sad he was gone.
>
> Thanks to this quick-thinking "escape strategy," I was no longer a "sore loser" but a grieving child, which felt like a more acceptable reason to be upset. Though I still didn't get Grandma to tuck me in, her attitude toward me shifted from accusation to sympathy. That moment marked the birth of an Escaper part in me—one that learned to fabricate or exaggerate the truth to dodge shame and protect my image. I realized it worked, and

I could pull it out of my pocket anytime I wanted to save face or avoid feeling shame.

At five years old, this seemed harmless, a simple reframing to sidestep discomfort. But what started as a quick fix became a habit, and over time, this Escaper didn't just bend the truth to soften small moments of vulnerability. It escalated into making more elaborate excuses and even telling outright lies, all in the name of saving face. I wasn't trying to deceive; I was trying to be seen in a positive light, stay in people's good graces and protect myself from feeling exposed. But protecting myself in this way sometimes meant distorting reality, avoiding accountability and creating unnecessary complications that, in the long run, caused far more damage than the initial moment of discomfort ever would have. What seemed like a small escape hatch as a child became a trap in adulthood, reinforcing my Inner Critic's belief that who I was—without an escape—was fundamentally problematic.

Mapping the Effects of the Escaper

Here, we provide a set of narrative practice questions designed to help you explore the effects of your Escaper parts and gain a more comprehensive understanding of how these strategies operate. You'll likely have several different Escaper parts, each with its own way of avoiding discomfort or overwhelm. You can go through these questions more than once to connect with the various strategies your different Escaper parts use.

The Impact of the Inner Critic and Shame on Your Escapers

- How have you noticed the dialogue between your Inner Critic and Shame influencing your behavior and feelings?
- Can you identify specific instances where this internal conversation led to escape behaviors?

The Overfunctioning Escaper

- Consider the times you've engaged in overachieving, perfectionism, excessive caregiving or whatever your specific style of overfunctioning looks like.
- When did this version of an Escaper come about?
- What approval, recognition or affection were you seeking?
- Reflect on the underlying belief that your worth needs to be earned. How has this belief impacted your sense of self-worth and satisfaction?

The Underfunctioning Escaper

- Reflect on moments of zoning out, numbing or indulging in distractions.
- How have these activities served as a refuge from reality for you?
- When did this version of the Escaper come about?
- How can you tell when you're genuinely decompressing versus using these behaviors to avoid your Inner Critic and Shame?

Aggression as an Escaper Response

- In what ways have your Escaper parts tried to relieve inner distress by turning the Inner Critic outward?
- Have you noticed moments when judgment, blame or even belittling others has served as a way to avoid your own discomfort or vulnerability?
- How and when does this typically happen?
- Do you have Escaper parts that use high-adrenaline, thrill-seeking behaviors or other risky actions to try to cope with inner pain or discomfort? If so, how do they do this?
- Alternatively, have you turned aggression inward, engaging in self-harm behaviors?

- What emotions or situations typically trigger these self-aggressive responses in you?
- What are the origins of these parts?

Impact of Escapers

- How have your Escaper parts (whether overfunctioning, underfunctioning or aggressive) affected your relationships with others?
- How have these Escaper parts impacted your relationship with yourself, your life and the decisions you make?
- Can you identify ways in which trying to escape has amplified your suffering or led to different forms of distress?
- Conversely, in what ways have these escape strategies helped?

Taking It In and Taking a Stand

Whatever you feel as you take in the scope of your Escapers' influence, it's welcome. Allow yourself, just for a moment, to acknowledge the impact these Escaper parts have had. It's important to let yourself feel the discomfort or regret over what's happened—not to dwell in it, but to face it. Taking a stand means recognizing the cost of your Escaper parts: the ways they've limited your presence, your integrity, your connection or your momentum. It means deciding not to keep looking away—even if you don't yet know what change will look like. Taking a stand begins with the willingness to want something different.

Moments of Power over Your Escapers

One way to shift your relationship with an Escaper is to notice the times when you were able to do something different—when you interrupted its typical momentum or made a choice that didn't follow the usual escape route. These moments may be

small, but they reveal something important: Sometimes, you've had your own power in relation to the Escaper.
- Are there moments when you felt the urge to escape but chose not to? What helped you stay with yourself in those moments?
- Can you recall times when you noticed an Escaper pattern starting and made a different choice? What was the impact of that choice?
- Are there areas of your life—certain relationships, routines or roles—where certain Escapers show up less often? Why do you think that is?

Externalizing Your Escapers

Now, let's focus on further externalizing your Escaper parts. Just as you did with the Inner Critic and Shame parts, you'll externalize and play with your Escapers to create more distance, gain perspective and increase your sense of agency in how you relate to this part. Go through these questions for one Escaper part at a time.

Characterization

- If your Escaper had a physical form, what would it look like? What color, shape and size is it?
- If your Escaper were a character or object, who or what would it be?
- Imagine, describe, draw or artistically represent its appearance, size or any distinguishing features.

Size and Distance

- Imagine placing your Escaper in the farthest corner of the room. How does that feel?
- Now, picture it outside the room entirely. What changes do you notice in yourself?

- If your Escaper appears larger than you, try shrinking it down. How does this affect its influence?

Genre Shift

- If your Escaper were in a movie, what genre would it be—an action-adventure movie, a sci-fi or fantasy epic, or a fast-paced thriller?
- Try "changing the channel" on your Escaper. How would it appear in a different genre?
- Visualize your Escaper as an animated character. How does this change your perception of it?

Voice Alteration

- What does the Escaper's voice sound like?
- Play with changing the pitch, tone and accent of your Escaper and notice if and how that feels different.

How Your Shame Triangle Parts Instigate Each Other

Now that we've explored the individual roles of the Inner Critic, Shame and the Escaper, it's time to examine how they interact. These parts don't just operate in isolation—they fuel and reinforce each other in a self-perpetuating loop. The Inner Critic's attacks stir Shame, which then provokes the Escaper to manage its distress. In the short term, the Escaper might provide some relief, momentarily soothing Shame or assuaging the Inner Critic, but when the Escaper's strategies go on too long or spiral out of control, they often backfire, leading to even harsher self-criticism or worse emotional discomfort. The overachieving Escaper eventually burns out, proving the Inner Critic right. The numbing Escaper procrastinates too long, resulting in Shame

feeling even worse. Each part has a way of kicking off the cycle or keeping it in motion. Consider the following questions:
- Which part in your Shame Triangle tends to activate first? Is there a predictable starting point—Inner Critic, Shame or Escaper—or does it depend on the situation?
- When your Inner Critic attacks, how does Shame respond? Does it absorb the criticism immediately, fight back or shut down?
- How do your Escapers try to intervene? Do they jump in to soothe the Shame, avoid discomfort or silence the Inner Critic?
- How long does the Escaper's strategy work before the cycle starts again? Does the numbing, distracting or overfunctioning actually bring relief, or does it eventually lead to more self-criticism or shame?
- If one Escaper's tactic doesn't work, does it switch to another Escaper part—going from overfunctioning to numbing, for example?
- Can you think of a time when you became aware of the cycle as it was happening? Did you do anything differently as a result of that awareness?

Δ

This chapter has been about raising your awareness of your Shame Triangle (or Triangles!). By mapping it out, you've taken an essential first step—a leap, really. The Shame Triangle thrives in the shadows, in unconscious repetition. But as you bring it into the light—identifying its origins, effects and strategies—you disrupt its automatic hold over you. You begin to step out of old, inherited scripts and into a space where the story can start to change. As you come to understand these parts more clearly, you no longer have to fear or fight them. They lose the power to take over in the ways they once did. This is the beginning of that shift.

CHAPTER 3
SHAME TRIANGLE ORIGINS AND TRIGGERS

In this chapter, we take a step back and examine where the Shame Triangle comes from and what keeps it active. Understanding both its origins and its triggers is essential to transforming it. By illuminating the cultural and relational forces that shaped the Shame Triangle, we can see how it's woven from threads far larger than our individual experiences. But knowing its roots is only half the journey. We also need to recognize what sparks the Shame Triangle in our day-to-day lives—the specific situations, interactions or inner shifts that set it in motion. When we identify these triggers, we gain the power to pause and choose a different path, rather than defaulting to old survival patterns.

Where Does the Shame Triangle Come From?

It's easy to believe the Shame Triangle is something that arises from within, a reflection of our own failings or proof that something is inherently wrong with us. All three parts—the Inner Critic, Shame and the Escaper—share this belief. Each one is convinced that the problem starts with you. That's the core logic of the Triangle itself, so it's easy to get caught inside their reasoning. But it isn't the full story. At its root, the Shame Triangle isn't simply a product of your personality or choices; it's a response to relational harm. It takes shape based on how we are treated by others, especially early on. Whether through criticism, neglect, conditional love or outright rejection, our early relationships teach us what is acceptable, lovable and worthy—and what is not. These messages don't just come through explicit lessons, but are also embedded in how caregivers responded to our emotions, the approval or disapproval we received, and the behaviors that earned us belonging or exclusion. Over time, we internalize these interpersonal experiences, shaping the roles of the Inner Critic, Shame and Escaper long before we have language for them.

But our Shame Triangle didn't start with the adults in our lives, either. Much like the Drama Triangle discussed in chapter 1, the Shame Triangle's origins are not personal. The beliefs our caregivers passed down came from the families they were raised in, the cultures they belonged to and the societies that shaped their worldviews. Culture, religion and society define what is right, who belongs and what it means to be worthy. These ideas shape how parents raise their children, how friends and colleagues interact, how we pursue education and careers, how we love and form relationships, and ultimately, how we judge ourselves and others.

For example, productivity culture's push to always do more conditions us to feel worthless when we slow down. Religious teachings around sin or purity can turn ordinary human desires into sources of shame. And the legacies of colonialism and slavery continue to perpetuate harmful stereotypes and systemic inequalities, reinforcing damaging beliefs about who belongs and who does not. Some of these messages are loud and explicit. Others are quieter, absorbed through everyday life. For example, a child sees their parent push through exhaustion, hears teachers praise students who never ask for help, and watches characters in movies and shows who are rewarded only when they appear selfless, high-achieving or emotionally detached. Over time, these cultural narratives imprint themselves onto our sense of self, shaping what we believe to be true about our worth. By understanding these broader contexts, we can begin to see how the Shame Triangle is not a reflection of our personal failings or deficiencies, but a product of the social messages we've been taught.

Below is a list of some cultural, social and historical narratives that create and reinforce our Shame Triangle parts. While this list is extensive, it's not exhaustive, so please identify any other influences that resonate with your specific life experience. As you read through these examples, take note of which of these cultural, social and historical factors have influenced the creation of your Shame Triangle.

Religious Doctrines

Teachings like original sin, sexuality as spiritual impurity, divine judgment, eternal damnation and karma as punishment for past misdeeds can create deep-seated beliefs that human nature is inherently flawed. We are seen as born corrupted, requiring divine salvation for redemption. Shame internalizes this sense of impurity, while the Inner Critic tracks moral "failures." Escapers may cope by driving us to pursue spiritual perfection, embrace extreme piety or reject faith entirely to escape the burden of guilt.

Capitalist Ideologies

Capitalist ideologies center productivity, profit and efficiency as measures of human value. In this system, worth is tied to output and rest is often seen as indulgent or lazy. We're taught to optimize ourselves—our time, energy and even our identities—for performance. This creates a relentless pressure to do more, achieve more and never slow down. Shame internalizes the belief that rest, stillness or prioritizing personal well-being signals weakness or lack of ambition. The Inner Critic echoes this, demanding constant productivity and shaming any moment of pause as laziness or failure. Escapers may overfunction by driving us into workaholism, using busyness to outrun feelings of inadequacy or avoid deeper needs. Others may underfunction by pushing us to collapse into exhaustion and numb out to escape the burnout cycle. Many of us move between these two Escapers, which push us to the brink, then retreat into shutdown, caught in a loop of overdrive and disconnection.

Legacies of Colonialism and Slavery

Racism, xenophobia, classism and the generational trauma of slavery linger in the body and psyche, shaping identity, belonging and self-perception, and convincing marginalized individuals they must overperform to be valued. Shame internalizes societal dehumanization, manifesting as a sense of unworthiness, hyperawareness of how we are perceived or an inherited fear of punishment for stepping out of line. This fear can manifest as feeling like an outsider in professional, academic or social spaces, believing success and/or acceptance require constant overperformance, or carrying an inherited sense of unworthiness due to generational marginalization. The Inner Critic reinforces these burdens, tracking every misstep as evidence of inadequacy or fueling hypervigilance to avoid judgment. Escapers may overfunction by making us strive for perfection, overwork to disprove stereotypes or assimilate at the cost of personal identity. Others may underfunction by telling us to disengage from opportunities that feel exclusionary, suppress our voice in spaces where we anticipate bias or numb the pain of systemic injustice through avoidance behaviors. Some of us oscillate between these two Escapers—overworking to break generational cycles, yet feeling guilt or futility when the weight of history proves impossible to outrun.

Individualism

This way of thinking glorifies self-sufficiency, making dependence or emotional needs shameful. The Inner Critic berates us for seeking support, while Escapers overfunction to prove independence or withdraw entirely from relationships. Rugged individualism discourages reflection, grief and emotional integration, demanding we "just move on."

Ableism

An ableist worldview creates unrealistic expectations of physical and mental abilities. Shame internalizes limitations as personal failures, and the Inner Critic harshly compares us to "normal" standards. Escapers may overcompensate by pushing us beyond our limits or avoiding situations that might expose our vulnerabilities, both actual and perceived.

Ageism

Cultural biases against both youth and older adults create shame around failing to meet age-related expectations. Young people are often dismissed as inexperienced or irresponsible, while older adults face pressures to remain productive or "age gracefully." The Inner Critic internalizes these judgments, making youth feel unqualified and elders feel obsolete. Escapers may overfunction, telling us we must constantly prove our worth—young people striving for credibility, older adults resisting signs of aging—or underfunction by making us withdraw from opportunities and relationships to avoid rejection.

Patriarchy

Patriarchy is a social system in which power and value are centered around masculinity, typically privileging men—especially cisgender, heterosexual men—while devaluing traits associated with femininity or emotional expression. Within this framework, rigid gender roles dictate who we should be and what parts of ourselves must be suppressed to meet societal expectations. This system marginalizes traits and identities that deviate from dominant norms, embedding shame in those who don't conform. We internalize the fear of being "too much"—too emotional, too assertive, too soft, too ambitious—or "not enough"—not strong enough, not attractive enough, not successful enough. The fear creates a chronic tension between authenticity and acceptability. The Inner Critic leverages this tension, punishing any deviation from traditional gender norms, policing self-expression and reinforcing the belief that worth is tied to how well one performs their assigned role. Escapers may overfunction by compelling us to strive to embody an idealized version of masculinity or femininity—overachieving to prove competence, repressing vulnerability to appear strong or sacrificing personal needs to meet expectations. Others may pressure us to rebel, withdraw or swing between both extremes, caught in an exhausting cycle of resistance and self-doubt.

Heteronormativity and Cisnormativity

These norms assume and enforce a narrow definition of what it means to be "normal" in terms of gender and sexuality, often defaulting to straight, cisgender identities. If we fall outside this frame, we are pressured to hide, mask or split off parts of ourselves to fit in. The result is a deep sense of shame and alienation for being "different." Our Shame parts can hold internalized homophobia, transphobia or biphobia, turning these cultural messages inward and compounding the pain of not fitting in.

The Inner Critic may enforce silence or secrecy, shaming desires or identity. Escapers might force us to compartmentalize, lead double lives or avoid intimacy altogether. Others may push us to try to "pass" to stay safe, meticulously managing how we present in different settings. Even those of us who are cis or straight (or both) may internalize these norms, unconsciously suppressing our own fluidity, softness or queerness in order to belong.

Classism and Socioeconomic Hierarchies

Classism is a system of inequality that ranks people based on income, wealth, education and social status—privileging those with economic power while devaluing those with fewer resources. Socioeconomic hierarchies shape how worth, intelligence and capability are perceived, often tying self-worth to financial success. As a result, economic struggles can feel like personal failings rather than the product of systemic barriers. The Inner Critic shames financial instability, equating it with laziness, irresponsibility or inadequacy. Escapers may drive us to overwork to gain a sense of security or value, pushing ourselves beyond our limits. Others may make us disengage from anything related to money—avoiding financial conversations, opportunities or responsibilities to escape the stress and shame tied to our circumstances.

Beauty Standards and Body Image Ideals

Beauty standards are culturally constructed ideas of what bodies and appearances are considered attractive, often shaped by media, consumerism and systems of power that uphold narrow, exclusionary ideals. These standards tend to favor youth, thinness, whiteness, able-bodiedness and other traits that marginalize diverse forms of beauty. Internalized, they distort our sense of self-worth, embedding the belief that attractiveness determines value.

Shame can convince us that our worth is tied to meeting these impossible ideals, making us feel unlovable or unattractive if we don't measure up. It often manifests more specifically: comparing oneself obsessively to idealized images, feeling unlovable or unworthy of desire, or developing a hyperawareness of perceived flaws. The Inner Critic amplifies these insecurities, scrutinizing every imperfection. Escapers may overfunction by encouraging extreme dieting, excessive exercise or cosmetic procedures in pursuit of unattainable perfection. Others may underfunction by telling us to avoid mirrors, social events or intimacy, or to numb our distress through comfort eating, compulsive shopping or digital filters that distort our self-perception.

Academic and Professional Achievement Pressures

These pressures stem from cultural and institutional systems that equate success with constant productivity, intellectual performance and outward accomplishments. From an early age, many of us are conditioned to believe that our value lies in how much we achieve, how smart we appear or how well we perform in school and work. Shame internalizes this belief, turning natural struggles into perceived failures. The Inner Critic tracks performance, comparing our achievements to those of others and fueling imposter syndrome. Escapers may overfunction by driving us to become perfectionists, work excessive hours or obsessively collect credentials to prove our worth. Others may underfunction by compelling us to procrastinate out of fear of falling short, self-sabotage to avoid potential failure or disengage from ambition altogether to escape the pressure of constant evaluation.

Consumerism and Materialism

Consumerism is a cultural system that encourages constant buying and accumulation of goods, while materialism links personal value to what one owns or displays. These forces shape the belief that success, happiness and even identity can be measured by possessions, lifestyle or financial status. Shame internalizes this message, creating the sense that having more means being more. This belief can manifest as insecurity when we can't keep up with trends, embarrassment over financial limitations or a fragile sense of self tied to material success. The Inner Critic reinforces these beliefs by comparing our home, appearance or status to those of others, stirring feelings of inadequacy or exclusion. Escapers may overfunction by encouraging us to chase status symbols, compulsively shop for validation or overwork to sustain a certain image. Others may underfunction by making us avoid financial realities, feel paralyzed by money-related stress, or numb our distress through impulse spending or complete disengagement from material aspirations.

Substance Use Culture

Substance use culture refers to the normalization, and often glamorization, of using alcohol, drugs or other substances to regulate emotions, avoid discomfort or foster social connection. In many environments, emotional distress is treated as something to be not felt or expressed, but numbed. Intimacy is often forged not through emotional presence, but through lowered inhibitions—bonding over shared intoxication rather than genuine connection. Shame absorbs the message that real connection requires performance, not authenticity, and that needing help to manage emotions is a personal failure. It can leave people feeling flawed for struggling to connect without a substance or for needing relief at all.

The Inner Critic plays a double role here. It may push our Escapers toward substances in the first place—insisting we need to relax, lighten up or keep it together—but then it turns around and berates us afterward. It shames us for using what it once suggested, calling us weak, out of control or broken. Meanwhile, Escapers may seek relief from the Inner Critic and Shame by compelling us to drown out our pain, anxiety or disconnection with substances. Some Escapers overfunction by helping us hold up a high-achieving or socially seamless exterior while secretly relying on substances to cope. Others underfunction by letting us withdraw into addiction, numbing ourselves to avoid facing our pain.

Instant Gratification Culture

Instant gratification culture prioritizes speed, convenience and immediate results. In this environment, discomfort is seen as a problem to eliminate and we're conditioned to expect quick fixes for complex challenges, from mental health to success. Shame internalizes the belief that struggle means failure and that if growth isn't fast or effortless, something must be wrong with us. The Inner Critic fuels this belief by demanding immediate progress, comparing our path to others' highlight reels, and shaming any delay, plateau or setback. Escapers may overfunction by pushing us to chase quick wins—seeking hacks, shortcuts or constant stimulation to feel productive or successful. Others may underfunction by making us avoid sustained effort, give up on long-term goals, or numb ourselves through impulsive choices, compulsive scrolling or fleeting pleasures. Many of us swing between these two Escapers—setting ambitious goals in bursts of motivation, then abandoning them when results don't come fast enough, trapped in a cycle of excitement, disappointment and self-blame.

Recognizing Internalization

As you explore your Shame Triangle parts throughout this book, we emphasize again and again how social and cultural forces shape not only our external realities but also our inner world. These dominant social narratives can become indistinguishable from our own inner voices, even if we don't consciously align with them. In narrative therapy, this process is called internalization—the point at which external messages become fused with our self-concept. The voice of a critical parent, the rigid rules of a religious upbringing or the silent pressures of societal norms all become part of our inner dialogue, masquerading as personal truth rather than external conditioning. Over time, we stop questioning these beliefs because they feel like "just the way things are."

Recognizing internalization changes how we see ourselves. It gives us a new vantage point—one that allows us to relate differently to both our inner experience and the external messages we've absorbed. Once you can see how these narratives have shaped your inner world, the next step is externalization—separating yourself from them so they no longer define you. This shift doesn't erase your experience, but it begins to dismantle the illusion that these stories are who you are. It opens the possibility of choosing what you want to carry forward, and what no longer belongs to you.

Instead of thinking *I am lazy and worthless because I took a day off*, externalization allows us to reframe: *The pressure to be constantly productive comes from a capitalist ideology that values output over well-being. My need for rest is natural and human, not a personal failing.* Instead of believing *I am the problem*, we begin to recognize *This problem originates within a larger system that shaped it.* Like stepping back from a single tree and realizing we're in a forest, we realize that what once felt like a private struggle is part of a much bigger picture. When we see the Shame Triangle as something absorbed from culture rather than something we *are*, we can begin to divest it of its harmful power, stop blaming ourselves and reclaim our sense of Self.

Reflection Questions

- What are some of the strongest self-judgments you experience? When you trace them back, can you identify where they may have originated—from family messages, cultural beliefs or societal expectations?
- How has your upbringing shaped your understanding of self-worth, success or identity? Do you notice ways these early influences still impact how you see yourself today?

- Can you recall a time when you felt shame or self-criticism? Looking beyond your personal reaction, what larger forces—such as gender roles, beauty standards, racism or work ethic ideals—might have contributed to that feeling?
- Where do you see the Shame Triangle reflected in the world around you—whether in media, workplaces, family dynamics or social norms? How do these external patterns shape your internal experience?
- Think of a self-judgment you often struggle with. If you were to externalize it, how would you rewrite the story? How might you challenge or reframe this belief in a way that frees you from its grip?

Shame Triangle Triggers

As you now have a better sense of the larger context from which the Shame Triangle arises, let's explore the external and internal stimuli that activate it in our daily life. Later, in chapter 7, we look at how Shame Triangle triggers affect the body by activating the nervous system's fight, flight, freeze and fawn responses.

Sometimes, the Shame Triangle is activated by something big—a breakup, a job loss, a betrayal. These major life events can act as powerful catalysts, pulling us into the grip of shame, self-criticism and escapism, and making it hard to stay grounded or clear. These triggers can also stem from other intense or overt situations, such as accidents, health diagnoses, the death of a loved one, significant life transitions, making a legitimate mistake or realizing we have caused harm. In these moments, the Shame Triangle takes over in a way that feels undeniable—the stakes are high, and the emotional toll is intense.

But not all triggers are so obvious. Sometimes, a Shame Triangle flare-up can be sparked by something much smaller: the way someone looks at you, the tone in their voice, an offhand comment, or even a particular smell or song that pulls up unexpected feelings. Because the trigger seems minor, our Inner Critic may jump in to shame us, accusing us of overreacting, being too sensitive or making things up. And sometimes, triggers don't even have to come from the outside—our imagination alone can summon them. Anticipating failure, imagining someone's disapproval or even envisioning a future mistake can be enough to activate the Shame Triangle. Whether large or small, real or imagined, these triggers can hook us fast—often before we even realize what's happening.

The Shame Triangle can be triggered by nearly any external or internal stimulus. In addition to those we've already named, here are some others:

External Triggers

- **Acute stressors**: Sudden challenges like receiving bad news, experiencing a conflict or facing a boundary violation can spark intense emotional responses.
- **Chronic stressors**: Ongoing struggles, such as financial strain, workplace difficulties or relationships that regularly ignore personal boundaries can gradually wear down our emotional resilience, making even minor stressors feel overwhelming.
- **Media exposure**: Social media, advertisements, TV shows and the news often promote unrealistic ideals of success, beauty and morality. Even neutral content can subtly plant seeds of comparison, self-doubt or inadequacy.
- **Environmental factors**: Living in an unsafe neighborhood, working in a toxic environment or navigating a chaotic home life can create a constant state of vigilance, making emotional responses more intense.
- **Unintentional reminders**: A particular smell, a familiar phrase or a setting reminiscent of past hurt can unconsciously revive old wounds.

- **Cultural and societal pressures**: Deeply ingrained messages about productivity, gender roles, body image and social status can influence self-perception, even in subtle ways.
- **Substance consumption**: Caffeine, sugar, artificial additives, alcohol and drugs can affect emotional regulation, making distressing thoughts or memories more difficult to manage.
- **Interpersonal rejection or exclusion**: Being ignored, left out, ghosted or dismissed can stir feelings of inadequacy and unworthiness.
- **Authority figures and power dynamics**: Encounters with bosses, teachers or other figures of authority—especially if they are critical, dismissive or withholding—can trigger the Shame Triangle.
- **Unmet emotional needs**: Feeling unseen, unappreciated or unsupported in relationships can create an underlying sense of emotional stress, making other stressors feel more intense.

Internal Triggers

- **Past experiences replaying in your mind**: Painful memories, even those long behind you, can resurface unexpectedly, bringing back emotional intensity as if the event were happening again.
- **Future anxieties**: *What if I embarrass myself? What if I fail?* Anticipating potential failure or judgment can initiate emotional distress preemptively, even if nothing has happened yet.
- **Physiological shifts**: Hunger, lack of sleep, hormonal fluctuations, medication side effects and certain substances can heighten emotional sensitivity and impact mental clarity.

- **Certain feelings and thoughts:** Strong emotions like frustration, loneliness, helplessness or even excitement can unexpectedly stir up the Shame Triangle.
- **Conflicting internal beliefs:** When personal values clash with external expectations—such as wanting to rest but feeling guilty about not being "productive"—it can create inner tension and self-judgment.

The Trouble with Positive Events

Many of us have a hard time welcoming moments of joy, success or even simple playfulness. As children, we might have been censored for laughing too loudly or told to "settle down" when we got too excited. Maybe in a moment of feeling proud about an accomplishment, we were told not to get a big head, or our expression of pleasure was frowned upon as indulgent. Or perhaps you heard phrases like "You should be grateful for what you have" not as a genuine invitation to appreciate your life, but as a weaponized way to silence your need, making it feel wrong to want more. Sexuality is also a source of shame. Many of us grew up absorbing messages that sexual desire was something to get rid of or feel guilty about. We might have been told certain feelings were inappropriate, that our bodies were gross or sinful, or that our curiosities made us bad or unworthy. Over time, this conditioning taught us that pleasure—whether emotional, physical, or sexual—is dangerous. That feeling too much, wanting too much or allowing ourselves to fully enjoy something will inevitably lead to punishment, rejection or regret.

So, when good things happen, we can find ourselves containing them, bracing ourselves for the fallout. This is why even positive experiences can destabilize you into a disorienting Shame Triangle spiral. Receiving a promotion at work might flood you with an inexplicable sense of impostor syndrome, as if you suddenly don't deserve the acknowledgment and everyone will discover you're a fraud. A new romantic relationship that begins beautifully could unleash latent insecurities, causing you to question whether you're worthy of love or fear that you'll inevitably lose it or mess it up. Celebrations like birthdays or weddings can ignite a rush of self-consciousness, intensifying our doubts about not living up to expectations. Even in moments of positive sexual connection, past conditioning may resurface, making it difficult to be present and causing Shame to take over where passion, intimacy or enjoyment could be. These counterintuitive moments—where something good unsettles your emotional balance—reveal the intricate and unpredictable ways in which the Shame Triangle can be triggered.

Jessica here!

This is precisely what happened to me during an important moment in my late twenties. I was in a two-year socially engaged Buddhism program and at our last in-person retreat, participants were invited to lead mini-workshops to share their unique expertise with their peers. I decided to teach a class on the Drama Triangle. By all external measures, my workshop went well. My peers gave positive feedback. People engaged with the exercises and shared that the workshop was insightful and beneficial for them. Objectively, I had every reason to feel good about it.

But despite this success, as the day continued, I found myself slipping into an unexpected Shame Triangle spiral. While attending my peers' workshops afterward, I found it nearly impossible to stay present. My Inner Critic had already started picking apart my performance—questioning my clarity, tone and delivery. At the same time, Shame had me scanning the room, trying to gauge whether people were more engaged in these sessions than in mine. Had I been clear and compelling enough? Did I measure up to the other presenters? Were people genuinely interested in what I had shared, or were they just being nice? Instead of being fully present and supporting my peers during their presentations, I was trapped in my own nightmare of self-doubt and comparison. Each time I caught myself drifting into my Shame Triangle stories, I'd attempt to refocus on the presentation at hand, only to further berate myself for being so self-absorbed.

By the time all of the workshops were over and the entire group reconvened in the meditation hall, my Inner Critic had reached full volume: *That was a disaster. You made such a fool of yourself.* Shame's resulting embarrassment and urge to disappear was so overwhelming, it became physical. I was dizzy and nauseous. My body felt heavy, as if gravity had intensified just for me. I couldn't sit up like everyone else—I needed to lie down. Fortunately, the setting allowed for some camouflage in that lying down with meditation cushions wasn't completely out of place, which enabled me to feign engagement in a "lying down" meditation to mask my turmoil. To further maintain appearances, my Escaper fabricated an excuse to those immediately around me about spontaneous back pain, saying it required me to do the meditation lying down, all while I was actually immobilized by an internal warzone, effectively playing dead to the world around me.

But the worst part wasn't just how harsh my Inner Critic had become—it was where it eventually aimed. Instead of stopping at my performance, it attacked my deepest sense of purpose: *You're not meant to do this. You don't have what it takes to help people. You should abandon this path before you embarrass yourself further.* My Inner Critic went for the jugular with this one, targeting what was most precious to me—my sense of purpose to be a positive support in this world—hammering me with the idea that I lacked what it really takes to make a difference in life. The weight of these words pressed down so hard that even standing up felt impossible.

As I lay there, stuck, my Escaper scrambled for exits: *Should I leave the retreat? Fake a family emergency? Escape to my dorm room?* But every escape route felt like another failure, further proof of me being a loser. What was happening to my body was so intense I thought I must be coming down with something, but that something was a Shame Triangle sickness, not an actual cold.

Despite my efforts to appear unaffected, one of the lead teachers sensed my distress and came over to check on me during a break. I cautiously admitted that I felt horrible despite knowing my presentation had gone well. He kindly suggested that what I was experiencing might be likened to the swing of a pendulum where my bold step to lead a discussion, especially among older seasoned speakers, had been an expansion beyond my comfort zone, so naturally, a contraction followed. He believed this act of stretching myself led to an opposite contraction and inward recoil, and my embarrassment wasn't proof of failure, but rather the aftershock of growth. I appreciated this perspective. His words helped, and even though they didn't erase the Shame Triangle knockdown I was in, they gave me more context. Even with his insights, I remained altered for the rest of the day. I felt hungover from the experience—exhausted, foggy, drained. It took time for my body and mind to recover from the sheer force of the Shame Triangle impacting me this severely.

This wasn't the worst Shame Triangle takedown I'd ever experienced, nor was it the last, but it was the first time I fully grasped how something positive could detonate an extreme Shame Triangle episode. No actual failure or humiliation had occurred. In reality, I had succeeded. Yet internally, it felt as if I had been booed off stage and ejected from the temple. The contrast between my internal lived experience and objective reality was staggering—and frankly, dangerous. What if I hadn't been able to wake up from that nightmare? What if I had taken it as truth and walked away from something I was meant to do? The experience made one thing crystal clear: The Shame Triangle isn't just a crappy voice in our head or a painful feeling. It can hijack the entire system, including the body, leaving us physically incapacitated—and it can do so even when things go right.

Reflection Questions

- What types of seemingly small or neutral events tend to trigger your Shame Triangle? Are there any patterns in the words, actions or environments that set it off?
- How does the media you consume impact your sense of self-worth? Do certain platforms, messages or comparisons leave you feeling inadequate? How do you respond when this happens?
- Are there specific physiological factors—such as foods, substances, sleep disturbances or hormonal changes— that make you more vulnerable to a Shame Triangle reaction? What adjustments could help you build more emotional resilience?
- Identify one chronic stressor in your life. How does this ongoing tension wear down your ability to cope? In what ways does chronic stress make you more sensitive to seemingly small triggers?
- Consider times when you've been caught in a "What if...?" spiral. How do imagined scenarios stir up shame or self-criticism? What strategies can help you stay grounded in the present and prevent a full Shame Triangle activation?
- Have you ever experienced shame or self-doubt in response to something positive, like a compliment, success or new opportunity? What underlying beliefs about being unworthy, exposed or not fitting in might have been triggered?

Δ

The Shame Triangle is reinforced daily—through media, workplace culture, casual conversations and in our closest relationships. It shows up in our thoughts and plays out in our interactions so seamlessly that even after recognizing its origins and understanding how it gets triggered, detaching from it isn't always immediate. Because of this reinforcement, awareness alone is not enough. True transformation requires something more: a genuine shift in perspective.

This is where the Self comes in—not another part of the triangle, but the steady presence within you that can witness these patterns without being consumed by them. The Self is not at war with the Shame Triangle. Instead, it witnesses, understands, loves and ultimately, leads. Learning to access this aspect of yourself is the foundation for change. In the next chapter, we turn our attention toward this inner ground. Before we begin the work of dialoguing with our Shame Triangle parts, we must first establish a connection to the Self—the place within you that is already whole, capable and unwavering, no matter what your Shame Triangle parts try to tell you.

CHAPTER 4
THE SELF

> *Jessica here!*

I was twenty-six when I first consciously encountered a presence within me that I now recognize as Self. It happened during a mindfulness workshop, where the facilitator guided us in connecting with an inner dimension beyond the confines of our ego, personality, social roles or labels—an inner sanctum of awareness that transcends the shifting tides of personal identity. The facilitator described this awareness not as the thoughts or emotions we experience, but as the luminous space from which those thoughts and emotions arise. They invited us to engage with an awareness that observes the content of our minds without being entangled in it. The intent was to offer each of us a glimpse of our core being, beyond our constructed self.

The exercise began with a seemingly simple task to write down all the different identities that define who we are. My race, language, gender, sex, profession, relational roles, even physical features—each found its place on individual slips of paper. As the facilitator guided us, I picked up each piece of paper, one by one, connecting with that specific identity. I immersed myself in each specific quality, trait or role that defined who I was, feeling its weight and significance in shaping my self-understanding, perception and interactions. We were then guided to envision life stripped of each label, as if it no longer existed for us. What would that feel like and who would we be without it? Then we symbolically placed each paper down to represent the release of that label.

In this guided process, shedding some identities felt easy, even liberating, for me. The notion of releasing my race and ethnicities was relieving, inviting a freeing contemplation of a world where such distinctions either cease to exist or cease to create such conflict. Other identities felt harder to let go of, such as being a friend, daughter or lover. While I could envision parting with them, I felt grief imagining life without these aspects of myself. Others felt near impossible to release. I could imagine changing my gender, sex or language to something different, but it was difficult to imagine not having a language, gender or biological sex at all, leaving me to question, *Who or even what am I without these defining traits? What is it that truly makes me "me," or any of us human for that matter?* Then I wondered if I could even let go of being human as just another identity. The very notion of existence without these pillars of identity left me grappling with the fundamental question of selfhood.

However, as I continued with the process, something significant emerged. Beyond the myriad labels and roles that I had previously assumed were inherent elements of myself, an underlying awareness was present that recognized these different roles and aspects of me—an awareness that transcended all identities, thoughts and emotional states. It wasn't another part of me that was simply wiser than the rest. It was consciousness itself. I experienced an awareness that was clear, centered and unwavering amid life's constant changes and challenges. It was steadfast even as my thoughts and emotions ebbed and flowed. This awareness felt both intimately personal, as if it was the very core of who I am, and transpersonal, as if it was connected to the universal intelligence that animates all life. While I had previously brushed against this experience of Self through meditation or substance-induced altered states, this experience marked the first conscious recognition of its profound significance—the realization that this core awareness was both a sanctuary to abide in and a wellspring of vitality I could live from. This experience revealed a dimension of myself that had always been present but overlooked, offering a perspective that was both grounding—rooting me to the earth—and infinitely expansive, connecting me to the cosmos.

It was a big realization. But often big realizations in the context of a workshop or retreat don't stick and can be challenging to integrate when we go home. Additionally, as I shared in the introduction to this book, meditation and spiritual teachings are often separate from psychological ones, so it wasn't until my encounter with Internal Family Systems (IFS) years later that I could fully integrate this experience of Self I had in my mid-twenties with the transformative journey of inner parts work I undertook in my thirties. After discovering my own awareness in this workshop, I needed time before I could apply it to my growth path.

The concept of Self can be tricky to explain. It's both distinct and elusive, concrete and abstract. We can sense Self-energy in ourselves and others, yet it slips through the fingers of definition, much like when we try to describe intuition, awareness or energy. Science can map the brain states associated with Self-energy*, just as it does with emotions or meditative states,

---

* Recent neuroscience research has identified distinct neural correlates of self-awareness, showing patterns of brain activity that align with different states of self-referential consciousness and awake awareness (Arenander and Travis 2004). Other studies suggest that self-awareness operates as part of a broader neurobiological framework, encompassing self-regulation and self-transcendence, particularly in mindfulness practices (Vago and Silbersweig 2012). These findings highlight the complexity of Self—both measurable and ineffable, rooted in neural processes yet extending beyond them.

but these experiences cannot be fully encapsulated by quantitative measurements alone. Each person's experience of their Self-energy is unique. Some describe it as a force—tingling, electric, alive in the body. Others experience it as a deep, quiet stillness, an expansive presence that holds everything: emotions, inner parts and the energies of those around them. Spiritual practitioners sometimes recount peak experiences as their initiation into accessing their higher Self with cathartic releases, full-body tremors, nervous system shifts, or what they call "cosmic downloads"—sudden insights or realizations that feel like they arrive all at once, without being mentally worked out. For others, tuning into Self for the first time may be a more understated experience, as they feel Self-energy as something simple and subtle—a gentle presence, rather than a dramatic revelation. Whether it comes as a whisper or a thunderclap, it is always an opening, and all these are equally valid ways of connecting to the same inner awareness.

We've already emphasized that Self is the foundation of parts work. Without Self-energy, we risk engaging with our parts from a place of urgency, frustration or reactivity rather than curiosity and compassion. Many clients say, "I've done so much work on this issue already," or "I've tried everything with this part." But when we pause and examine who is truly leading the process, we often discover it's not the Self—it's another part, and no matter how well-intentioned, when parts try to lead, the work stalls.

This distinction is pivotal. Without Self-energy, the Shame Triangle becomes a maze. We try to find our way out, only to keep hitting dead ends. With Self-energy, we can finally step out of the maze. It creates the space to unblend from these parts, witness them without being overtaken, and engage with them from a place of understanding, rather than resistance. The challenge is that the Shame Triangle makes it difficult to access Self, yet only Self can transform it. When we are fully caught inside it, our perspective is limited to the parts driving it. We become so blended with them that their pain, fear and judgments feel like absolute reality, but when Self is present, we gain enough space to see these parts for what they truly are: wounds and protective strategies, rather than our core identity. From this place, real transformation becomes possible.

The Self in IFS

According to the IFS model, we all have different parts that help us navigate life. Manager parts keep us moving—handling responsibilities, showing up for work and maintaining our daily routines. Other parts carry pain, the weight of past experiences or the scars of marginalization and injustice. Then there are our protectors—the parts that step in to shield us from feeling too much, too fast. They work to keep us safe, to prevent us from looking bad, losing connection or jeopardizing our place in the groups we belong to. Their strategies—whether perfectionism, people-pleasing or staying small—are meant to protect us from what we fear the most. But sometimes, their efforts become so rigid that they block growth rather than support it, and over time, we can start to mistake their voices for the whole truth about who we are.

At the core of IFS is the concept of Self, or Self-energy—our true, unshakable essence, existing beyond the fears, wounds and agendas of our parts. The discovery of Self was a turning point in the development of IFS. Richard Schwartz (2021), the founder of IFS, first encountered Self in his clinical work. As he helped clients work with their parts, he noticed a pattern: When protective parts were asked to step back, something unexpected emerged. Clients described a presence that was calm, clear and unlike any of their usual internal voices. It wasn't another part with its own agenda—it was something deeper. When Schwartz asked clients to name what they were experiencing, they often struggled to put it into words, simply calling it "me." This presence was distinct from their pain and trauma, yet capable of holding and healing their wounded parts with a natural, effortless compassion. Even those with severe trauma histories had access to it, revealing that Self-energy was not something earned or developed—it was an innate aspect of being human. This realization reshaped the IFS model. Schwartz saw that no matter what someone had been through, their Self remained intact. It could be obscured but never destroyed. When someone struggled to access their Self, it wasn't because they lacked it but because their protective parts were blocking it, often out of fear that being in Self would make them vulnerable. Over time, Schwartz found that helping clients build trust with these protectors allowed Self to emerge more fully, creating the conditions for lasting healing.

To help people recognize when they are in Self, Schwartz identified eight qualities that naturally emerge in Self-energy: compassion, curiosity, calm, confidence, courage, clarity, connectedness and creativity. These qualities—often referred to as the "Eight C's of Self"—serve as signposts, helping us distinguish when we are in Self versus when a part is running the show.

Each of these C's reflects a different dimension of Self-energy:

- **Compassion**: A natural kindness and warmth toward ourselves and others, without judgment.
- **Curiosity**: A genuine openness to our inner world and the experiences of others, without needing to control or assume.
- **Calm**: A sense of inner steadiness, free from urgency or reactivity.
- **Confidence**: Trust in ourselves and in the process of healing, even when we don't have all the answers.
- **Courage**: The ability to face what we fear—whether within ourselves or in the world—without shutting down.
- **Clarity**: The capacity to see ourselves, others and our circumstances without distortion or the filters of our wounds.
- **Connectedness**: A deep sense of belonging—to ourselves, to others and to something greater.
- **Creativity**: The freedom to imagine new possibilities, unburdened by limiting beliefs or old patterns.

These qualities are not skills to develop or traits we must "earn"—they are inherent aspects of Self. However, certain parts can block access to them. For example, a hypervigilant part that expects danger may make it difficult to feel calm. A people-pleasing part may hold back curiosity, fearing that asking the wrong question could create a problem. A perfectionist part might override creativity, insisting that only flawless work is acceptable. But these blocks aren't barriers we should push through—they are invitations. Rather than forcing access to the Eight C's, we cultivate them by building trust with all our parts. As we listen to and work with them, we naturally create more space for Self-energy to emerge.

While trauma, mental health challenges and brain injuries can make it more difficult to access Self, our Self-energy is always present. For some of us, the journey to embody it is slow, requiring patience and practice—especially if we were never taught to recognize it. At first, Self-energy may feel unfamiliar or elusive, but as we learn to access it, we realize we are supported by an incredible resource within. This discovery can be both challenging and empowering: it requires unlearning old patterns, and it reveals that a healing, stabilizing presence is already within us. No matter where we come from or what we've been through, everyone has access to Self-energy and can learn to embody it.

For those with spiritual or religious perspectives, the experience of Self may already be familiar under different names, such as Buddha-nature, Atman, Eternal Oneness, Christ Consciousness or the divine spark. Across spiritual traditions, there is a recurring recognition of an inner essence that transcends the ego and connects us to something greater, whether it is seen as enlightenment, unity with the divine or the fundamental nature of reality. While IFS offers one way to connect with Self-energy, spiritual traditions provide another doorway, reinforcing the idea that this inner essence is not only real but universally accessible.

Self-Leadership

The primary goal of IFS is to cultivate Self-leadership, where our Self-energy becomes the guiding force in our lives, rather than letting our various inner parts lead the way. Ideally, the Self sits confidently in the driver's seat of our internal system, with our parts riding along as passengers—helpful companions, but not the ones at the wheel. Yet for many of us, the opposite often happens. Our wounded or protective parts take control, while Self is pushed to the backseat—or worse, locked away in the trunk, barely present at all. When these parts are in charge, we blend with their perspectives, losing sight of the fact that each part represents only a fragment of our experience, not the full picture. Self-leadership, in contrast, allows the Self to hold a panoramic view that no single part can offer. The Self can empathize with the truths and struggles of each part while also transcending their limiting beliefs and judgments. This broad perspective gives us access to greater clarity, wisdom and flexibility, helping us better navigate both our inner and outer worlds.

Being parts Led: left and center. Being Self Led: right.

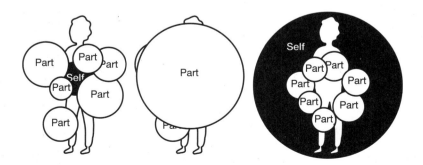

It's worth noting that some of our parts can carry a substantial amount of Self-energy. For instance, parts that embody our core values—like integrity, justice or kindness—can display qualities that feel very aligned with the Self. These parts may guide us toward actions that reflect our highest principles and longings. However, parts are not Self, and even if they express a lot of Self-energy, they can never fully replace it. And while some parts genuinely embody Self-energy, others may only mimic it. For example, a performer part may seem confident, but its confidence may depend on external validation rather than the deep trust that arises from Self. A visionary part may appear creative, but its creativity may be driven by urgency or pressure rather than the expansive, inspired quality of Self. The difference lies in the energy behind it, where Self-energy is effortless, without an agenda. When we are in Self, we don't need to push for calm; it simply arises. We don't have to force courage; it is already present. Compassion, too, flows naturally, and we don't have to manufacture it or try to be kind. This energy is what distinguishes Self from our parts: it is not reactive, performative or striving. It just is.

That said, while some parts may be cut off from Self-energy—disconnected by fear, burdens or past wounds—they are not permanently separated. As we engage in this work, building trust with our protective parts and bringing care to our wounded parts, something powerful happens: Parts that were once isolated begin to reconnect with Self. As they do, they don't just step aside for Self-energy—they become infused with it. Over time, they soften, unburden and take on more of the Eight C's of Self. This is one of the most beautiful aspects of parts healing—not only do we access more Self-energy, but our parts express more Self-energy, too.

So how do we know whether we're operating from Self or from a part? Consider two key qualities: the level of perspective, and the underlying mode of action. Parts are typically oriented around *doing*—they have specific roles, agendas and tasks they're trying to accomplish, whether those tasks are avoidant, lofty or well-intentioned. No matter how wise or visionary a part may be, its view is still shaped by its role—it sees through a particular lens, often limited to the situation at hand. Self, on the other hand, is not trying to do—it is rooted in *being*. It doesn't have an agenda. Its presence is open and inclusive. When we're in Self, we can take in many perspectives at once without becoming entangled with any single perspective. We can sense the emotions of our parts without being swept away by them. This is the hallmark of Self-leadership: the ability to hold the full complexity of our inner world with presence, clarity and care—and to respond from that grounded center rather than from reactivity or habit.

Speaking *for* Our Parts Instead of *from* Them

An essential practice for being Self-led in IFS is learning to speak *for* our parts rather than *from* them. Speaking from a part means we are blended with that part's perspective, seeing only through its lens and temporarily losing access to Self-leadership. Our words and actions are dictated by the part's emotions and beliefs, often without us realizing it. For example, if an anxious part takes over, we might find ourselves catastrophizing or ruminating, convinced that the worst-case scenario is inevitable. We might blurt out, "This is never going to work out. I'm doomed to fail," fully absorbed in the anxious part's fear. In these moments, we're not in Self; we're merged with the part, speaking as it.

When we're blended with a part, especially one from the Shame Triangle, it often feels like we *are* the part because its impulses drive our thoughts, emotions and behaviors. We don't just feel anxious, ashamed or critical—we grab a drink, cancel plans, sign up for another workshop, micromanage or lash out at someone we love. These actions are often so familiar and reinforced that they feel like "just who we are." But in truth, they're being driven by a part. As we strengthen our ability to unblend, we can begin to notice the part's impulse before we act on it and in that moment, we gain the power to respond rather than react.

However, when we speak from a part without recognizing it, we risk slipping into its emotional reality, which can distort communication and create conflict. This often shows up as blaming, shaming, "shoulding," exaggerating, accusing, catastrophizing or mislabeling ourselves and others. Because we are fused with the part, we speak as though its perception is the whole truth and nothing but the truth. This fusion can compel us to use reactive language, defaulting to "you" statements rather than "I" statements—telling others what they did, what they meant or how they made us feel, instead of owning our own experience. This type of language usually creates defensiveness in the other person and makes it harder to engage in meaningful dialogue.

On the other hand, speaking for our parts means we remain centered in Self while acknowledging the part's emotions and perspective. Instead of being fused with the part, it's as if we are standing beside it, translating its experience rather than letting it take over. The Self's expansive awareness allows it to hold space for the part's fears, needs and beliefs while also guiding us toward wiser, more balanced responses. For example, if an anxious part arises, instead of saying, "This is never going to work out," we might say, "I notice my anxious part is really activated right now and worrying about all the ways this could go wrong." This shift creates space for a broader perspective. From this place, we can also then reality-check whether the anxiety is based on an actual or hypothetical danger, soothe the part and explore solutions rather than reacting impulsively.

Learning to differentiate between speaking from a part and speaking for a part can be a turning point in how we relate to others. When we speak from a part, our words often carry blame, judgment or defensiveness, evoking others' protective parts and escalating conflict. But when we speak for a part, we create an opening for understanding. For instance, we might say, "I'm noticing my manager part is feeling anxious, and it's making me want to control things. I realize this isn't really about you. Can we take a pause and return to this conversation when I'm feeling more grounded?" By naming the part and its feelings, we take responsibility for our inner experience while also signaling that it's not the full story or a reflection of the other person. This helps to disarm defensiveness and invites the other to lean in instead of away.

Speaking for our parts also allows us to communicate needs and boundaries more effectively. Instead of reacting impulsively or making demands, we can express our truth in a way that invites collaboration and understanding. For example, rather than saying, "You never support me!" from a victim part that "feels" abandoned, we might say, "There's a part of me that's feeling very alone right now and needing some reassurance. Could we talk about that?" This approach fosters intimacy, trust and mutual respect—essential ingredients for deeper connection.

An important takeaway here is that when we speak for our parts rather than from them, we recognize that all parts—whether they bring pleasant or challenging emotions—have something valuable to share. Our work isn't to silence or control them, but to understand them, integrate them and help them heal so they can express their highest potential under the guidance of the Self. However, this goal doesn't mean we should always aim to unblend from our parts. Blending isn't inherently bad—it's a natural and sometimes necessary way of experiencing life. The goal isn't to keep parts at a distance, but to cultivate the discernment of when blending serves us and when it limits us. In some moments, being fully blended with a part is essential and beneficial. A rageful part might fight back in a moment of real danger, ensuring our survival. A hurt part might express raw emotion in a way that allows someone to truly see our pain—something a composed explanation could never convey. A tender part might bring us to tears at the sight of something beautiful, allowing us to fully take in the depth of a moment.

Sometimes, the path to unblending actually begins with blending. If a part has been ignored, silenced or exiled for years, it may first need us to fully allow it to express itself, to step into its shoes. In these cases, blending isn't a setback or a regression—it's a necessary step in our process of accepting a part and giving it permission to take up space, without rushing to separate from it. Once a part has been allowed to fully inhabit us, and be felt, expressed and experienced from the inside, unblending often becomes possible, not as a forced technique, but as a natural consequence of having made space for the part within us.

The key is awareness and choice. Some situations call for blending—getting lost in the flow of creativity, expressing deep love, grieving, or surrendering to joy and playfulness. In these moments, we don't need to step back; we can allow the part's presence to be fully felt. And even then, we might recognize that we are blended and choose to stay that way, embracing the experience. On the other hand, during difficult conversations, boundary-setting or moments of conflict, blending often leads to misunderstanding, escalation or reactivity. In these situations, speaking for our parts becomes most important.

The Self doesn't control our parts—it guides them. Like the conductor of an internal orchestra, the Self brings coherence, attunement and rhythm to the whole system. Each part has its own role to play, its own instrument to contribute. Some may have solo moments, while others play supporting roles. The goal isn't to silence any part but to harmonize them, ensuring that no single instrument drowns out the rest. The Self's role is to allow all parts to be heard while holding the broader vision of balance and connection. Learning to speak for our parts is a powerful practice—one that fosters Self-leadership, emotional intelligence and authentic connection not only within ourselves but also in our relationships with others.

Here are some examples illustrating the difference between speaking for a part versus from it.

Table 3. Speaking from Versus Speaking for a Part

Speaking from a Part	Speaking for a Part
"This is too much. I can't handle this."	"I notice that there's a part of me that feels scared and overwhelmed about this situation."
"I don't want to deal with this shit!"	"There is a part of me that wants to withdraw and protect myself."
"You never understand me, and I'm tired of it!"	"There's a part of me that feels angry because I feel misunderstood."
"If I don't do this perfectly, I'm a failure. I can't fail; it has to be perfect."	"I recognize that my perfectionist part is worried about making mistakes."
"I'm scared and alone; nobody cares about me!"	"I sense that my inner child part is feeling vulnerable and needs reassurance."
"I can't handle not knowing what's going to happen; it's driving me crazy!"	"I'm aware that my anxious part is feeling overwhelmed by uncertainty."
"I'm worthless; I'll never amount to anything."	"I notice that my critic part is being harsh because it's trying to protect me from failure."
"I have to take care of everyone else before myself; it's my duty."	"I sense that my caretaker part is feeling responsible for everyone's well-being."

A final point on why we are so jazzed about the concept and practice of Self-leadership is that it changes where we source our sense of Self. It challenges us to ask: Is our source of meaning, stability and fulfillment external or internal? So often, we look to others—partners, friends, family members or mentors—as the primary source of our happiness, healing or sense of purpose. We may unknowingly outsource our sense of Self, relying on external validation or relationships to fill emotional voids. This can lead to looking for others to complete us, believing that only through them can we feel whole, worthy or safe. While connection and support from others are essential, this dynamic can create dependency, leaving us vulnerable when external sources falter or change.

Being Self-led shifts this paradigm. It roots our sense of wholeness in something internal, something unshakable—our own Self. From this place, others in our lives become a complement to our inner foundation rather than the foundation itself. We can still receive love, help, wisdom and connection from those around us, but our wellspring of fulfillment, meaning and healing comes from within. This perspective doesn't just lead to more balanced relationships—it changes the way we experience life itself. Instead of feeling like we're at the mercy of external circumstances, we become anchored in something deeper, something that remains steadfast, no matter what is happening around us.

Reflection Questions

- How do you experience your own Self-energy? Are there particular activities, practices or moments when you feel most connected to it? How might you create more opportunities to access and embody Self-energy in your daily life?
- Reflecting on your own experiences, can you identify moments when your protective or wounded parts have taken over the driver's seat? How might these situations have been different if your Self-energy had been in the lead?
- Consider the qualities of Self-energy: compassion, curiosity, calm, confidence, courage, clarity, connectedness and creativity. Which of these qualities do you find easiest to access, and which ones feel more challenging? For the qualities that feel more difficult to access, which parts get in the way? What practices might help you strengthen your connection to these qualities?

- When you think about the difference between speaking from a part and speaking for a part, can you recall a recent interaction where you were speaking from a part? How could you have shifted to speaking for the part, and how might that have changed the outcome?
- What are some ways in which your parts may have contributed positively to your life, even if they initially seemed problematic? How can you honor these parts while also guiding them toward more constructive roles under the leadership of Self?

Exercises for Cultivating Self-Connection

Understanding Self as an embodied presence in our lives is one thing; learning how to access it in a reliable and sustainable way is another. Many people grasp the concept of Self-energy but struggle with applying it in moments of stress, reactivity or emotional overwhelm. To deepen our ability to lead from Self, we need practices that help us return to this state, strengthen our inner connection and stay attuned to Self-energy even in challenging situations.

In this section, we provide a variety of guided practices to support you in accessing and strengthening your relationship with Self-energy. While you may not resonate with all of them, we encourage you to approach each practice with an open mind and give each one a try at least once, since you may be surprised by the experiences that unfold. The journey of connecting with our Self is very personal. Some practices may feel like an instant fit, while others may take time to fully appreciate. Trying these exercises is essential for transforming the Shame Triangle and unlocking the deeper shifts that the rest of the book will guide you through. Embrace this process as an ongoing exploration and allow yourself to remain open to new experiences and insights along the way.

Discovering Your Awake Awareness Beyond Your Identities

This exercise is designed to guide you through a journey of disidentification similar to the one Jessica described at the beginning of the chapter to help you discover the aware presence that exists beyond your constructed identities. You will be guided through externalizing and temporarily letting go of the different ways you describe and identify yourself. This exercise is about recognizing the underlying awareness that exists beyond your parts. It's a practice of coming home to the foundational awareness that is your true nature. For this exercise, you will need a quiet, comfortable space, several slips of paper and something to write with.

Sit comfortably in a quiet space where you won't be disturbed. Take several deep breaths, centering yourself in the present moment.

Identify your identities. On individual slips of paper, write down at least ten of the various identities that define you (i.e., your different roles, relationships, attributes, etc.). Pick the identities that are most important to you or the ones that seem the hardest to be without. Place these slips of paper in front of you.

Pick up one piece of paper. Take a few moments to connect with that identity. Step into it fully. Reflect on what it means to you, how it defines you and how it shapes your life.

Imagine your life without this identity. If this way of identifying yourself didn't exist for you, what would that be like? How would you be the same or different? What would your sense of self and the world look and feel like? Who would you be?

Visualize and/or feel letting go of this identity. Place the slip of paper down, symbolizing the release of this part of you. Notice any feelings or sensations that arise. Some may bring relief, while others may feel uncomfortable.

Repeat with each identity. Continue this process with each slip of paper one by one, moving at your own pace.

After letting go of all the identities, sit quietly and bring your attention inward. Observe any thoughts, emotions or sensations that arise, without attaching to them. Tune into the awareness that is aware of all the parts and identities that you have connected with and let go of. Feel the presence of awareness itself. This is your consciousness, your awake awareness—the space in which all thoughts and identities appear and dissolve. Abide here as long as you'd like.

Call back your identities. When you're ready, you can call all these labels back to you. Imagine them returning. You can also let some stay released, if you prefer.

Gently return to your body. Return your attention to the space you are in. Open your eyes and look around, reconnecting with your body and the fullness of you, with this awareness and all your identities. Recognize that this awareness is always available to you, beneath the layers of identity. Bring it with you into the rest of your day.

The Universal Me Meditation

This exercise is meant to connect you with different universal qualities.

> **Jessica here!**

I first developed this Universal Me practice years ago when I realized that simply using positive affirmations or wishing to embody certain qualities wasn't as effective as directly experiencing them. Rather than praying for change as if who I wanted to be existed outside of me, something I needed to receive or be granted, I began inviting these universal qualities to flow through me—as if they were already available, already present within. Instead of asking for more courage, clarity or love, I would step into those qualities and let myself feel them as part of my being. This shift—from seeking to embodying—was transformative for me, and it's what makes this practice so powerful.

This exercise helped me realize that qualities like love, peace, beauty, humor and wisdom are traits that, yes, we can cultivate over time, but they are also universal forces that we can receive anytime. We don't have to chase, manufacture or struggle to maintain them—they are already present, available to flow through us when we allow it. While we can nurture these qualities within ourselves, we can also tap into them, letting them move through us, rather than believing we must generate them from scratch.

I first used this practice when I was nervous about a job interview. I wanted to show up as my most confident, personable and vibrant self—the ideal candidate for the job. Before the interview, I sat in my car and imagined connecting with the core of the earth, anchoring myself in something greater. Then, I visualized each of the qualities I wanted to embody rising up through that connection and flowing into me—filling me up and radiating outward. I didn't have to force myself to be confident or charming; I simply allowed those qualities to move through me. I wasn't striving or performing, I was just present, an open vessel for universal forces to move through. When the interview began, I noticed a shift. I felt more grounded and at ease. When I was asked questions, I didn't rush to impress—I responded with more clarity and honesty. I was comfortable naming what I knew and what I didn't. Something more authentic was speaking through me. That experience stayed with me. Since then, I've used this practice in countless moments—giving talks, going on dates, having difficult conversations, anytime I wanted to express my best, most resourced Self. And each time, it has made a difference.

I've also found that, as we progress in our parts work, this practice can be especially helpful for Shame parts. Our Shame parts often struggle to believe that we are certain ways, especially if we've never been that way before or only experienced it intermittently. For example, I once worked with a client whose younger Shame part believed she was ugly because everyone—including her parents—had told her so. She couldn't simply hear from Self that she was beautiful; that would have felt like a lie to her. But what we could do was help her connect to the universal quality of beauty itself. She didn't have to convince herself she was beautiful in the way she had been taught to define it—she could simply let beauty move through her and experience it, regardless of what she looked like then or now. This approach helped her feel a sense of worth and connection to something greater than her conditioned beliefs, creating space for healing in a way that compliments or self-affirmations alone never could.

Now let's try it...

Get comfortable. Sit tall or lie down in a relaxed position. Take a few deep breaths to ground yourself.

Connect to the earth. Imagine a cord of light or tree roots extending from the bottom of your body down into the earth's core. Feel yourself becoming anchored and supported.

Call in a quality. From this grounded connection, choose the first quality you want to receive—one that you want to embody right now. Say it to yourself: "I am love."

Let it fill you. Feel unconditional love flowing up from the earth and through your body, filling you completely. Allow that quality to move through every part of you—your body, your breath, your energy. Let it expand within you. Don't force anything. Just receive.

Move to the next quality. When you're ready, choose another quality. Breathe it in and repeat it to yourself as a simple affirmation:
- "I am peace." (Feel a deep stillness and calm settle within you.)
- "I am joy." (Feel your whole body and being smile, lit from within.)
- "I am strength." (Sense your inner power and resilience.)
- "I am beauty." (Feel yourself radiating the essence of true beauty.)
- "I am compassion." (Let warmth and tenderness open your heart.)
- "I am confidence." (Feel the quiet certainty of knowing who you are and what you bring.)
- "I am wisdom." (Connect to clarity and deep inner knowing.)

Continue feeling whichever qualities you want to experience and embody. Allow each one to fully flow through you and expand inside you. Really feel it, let it move through every cell and enjoy its presence.

Radiate outward. When you feel full, visualize these qualities shining from you.

Take a final deep breath. Rest in the feeling of your Universal Self. Return to this practice anytime. Repeat these affirmations and reconnect with this state whenever you need it throughout your day.

Unblending from a Part

This practice strengthens your ability to step in and out of a part's perspective, helping you develop psychological and energetic distance. We are not engaging in a conversation with the part yet—just practicing the act of unblending. Think of this exercise like doing reps at the gym: The more you practice unblending, the easier it becomes to shift back into Self-energy.

Find a quiet space. Sit comfortably and take a few deep breaths to center yourself.

Choose a part. Pick a part you'd like to practice unblending from. It might be one that has been particularly active or distressing lately, or it can be one that you think will be easy to practice with.

Bring awareness to the part. Notice any physical sensations, emotions or thought patterns connected to it.

Externalize it. Imagine or sense the part moving outside of you, as if it's now in front of you. You don't need to see it clearly—just experience it as something separate from you.

Notice what else is there. With the part outside of you, check in with what remains. Do you feel relief, spaciousness or calm? Or does something else arise—perhaps sadness, emptiness or another part beneath the surface? Just observe.

Step back in. Now, allow the part to return inside. Notice how it feels to be blended again.

Repeat the process. Externalize the part again. Let it step outside of you for a few seconds and then have it step back in again. Then externalize it once more. Take a few breaths and feel the separation from this part. Then invite it to step back in.

Getting to Know a Part

Now that you've practiced unblending, this exercise helps you deepen your relationship with a single part by creating a safe space for connection. This exercise is particularly useful when a part feels intensified, stuck or distressed.

Find a quiet space. Sit comfortably, close your eyes and take a few deep breaths to settle and center into your Self-energy.

Imagine a safe space. This could be a real place or a completely imagined environment—somewhere that feels grounding, protective and uniquely yours.

Invite a part forward. Choose a part that has been particularly active lately that you would like to talk with. Let it know you would like to connect with it (not get rid of it) and ask it to step outside of you for a few minutes so you two can talk. If any other parts are present, you can ask them to step aside for a few minutes while you focus on this one part.

Engage in dialogue. From the perspective of Self, gently ask the part:
- When did you come about in my life?
- What do you want me to know?
- What do you need?
- How can I best support you?

Listen with warm, open interest. Acknowledge whatever the part shares without judgment. Pay attention to any shifts in emotion, imagery or bodily sensations.

Reassure the part. Let it know that its voice matters and that you, as Self, are here to lead—not to ignore it or push it away, but to understand and support it.

Close with gratitude. Thank the part for showing up. Remind it that this safe space is always available and that you will return when needed.

Parts Around the Campfire

Now that you've practiced unblending from a single part, this exercise takes unblending a step further by unblending from multiple parts at once. Visualizing your parts gathered around a campfire allows you to more fully access Self-energy. This practice is especially helpful when you feel overwhelmed by the voices of too many parts speaking up at once and are struggling to find clarity.

Find a comfortable seated position and take a few deep breaths to ground yourself.

Visualize yourself in a peaceful forest clearing with a warm campfire in the center.

Tune into your parts and invite them forward. Notice various parts of yourself beginning to emerge and take a seat around the campfire.

One by one, externalize these parts fully, allowing them to step outside of you into the space around the fire. Breathe into any sense of lightness or spaciousness this creates within you.

Continue this process until all identifiable parts have been externalized, leaving you with a sense of pure, expansive Self-awareness.

Relax back into this state of Self-energy, allowing qualities like calm, compassion, clarity and courage to arise naturally.

Spend time simply being present with your parts while anchored in your Self. You can engage in internal dialogue if desired.

When you're ready, invite the parts back one by one, integrating them into your inner landscape.

Take some deep breaths and open your eyes, carrying your grounded Self-energy into your day.

Connecting with the Eight C's of Self

This exercise guides you through connecting with each of the Eight C's of Self—compassion, curiosity, calm, confidence, courage, clarity, connectedness and creativity. These qualities are already within you, but daily life and protective patterns can make them feel distant. By intentionally focusing on them, you strengthen your ability to access Self-energy more readily.

Find a comfortable seat and take a few deep breaths, settling into yourself. If it feels right, invite your parts to step back so you can fully embody Self-energy. There is no need to push them away; just let them know they are welcome to rest for now while you connect with these qualities.

Compassion: Bring to mind a moment when you felt genuine compassion for someone—a loved one going through difficulty, an animal in need or yourself during a challenging moment. Notice the warmth and care that arises within you. Feel this compassion expanding through your body, softening any tension, opening your heart. Let yourself rest in this feeling, allowing it to deepen your capacity for kindness and presence.

Curiosity: Think of a time when you felt truly curious—perhaps exploring a new place, learning about a subject that fascinated you or simply marveling at something in nature. Tap into that sense of open wonder. Shift your awareness to the present moment with that same gentle curiosity, noticing whatever thoughts, emotions or sensations arise without judgment, as if you're getting to know them for the first time.

Calm: Recall an experience that brought you deep peace—sitting by the ocean, being alone in nature or lying in bed in the quiet moments before sleep. Let that sense of ease fill you now, releasing tension from your body. Your breath slows. Your mind softens. You are still, present and at peace.

Confidence: Remember a moment when you felt strong and self-assured. It might have been during a challenge you faced, a time you spoke your truth or a moment of simply feeling comfortable in your own skin. Notice how confidence feels in your body—the way you stand, the way you move. Let this grounded assurance grow within you, knowing that your wisdom and inner resources are always available.

Courage: Think of a time when you or someone you admire acted with courage. Maybe it was standing up for what was right, stepping into the unknown or facing something difficult with an open heart. Feel that courage alive within you. It doesn't mean the absence of fear—it means moving forward despite it. Trust in your own resilience.

Clarity: Bring to mind a moment when your mind felt clear—maybe during a moment of insight when something finally clicked, in a meaningful conversation that shifted your perspective, or after releasing something you'd been carrying for too long. There was no confusion, just direct knowing. Imagine your mind now like a vast, clear sky—open, expansive and undisturbed. From this place, you can see your inner world and life's complexities with wisdom and understanding.

Connectedness: Remember a moment when you experienced deep connection—whether with a loved one, a friend, a community, the natural world or something greater than yourself. Notice the feeling of being truly met, seen or in sync—a sense of togetherness that reminds you that you're not separate, but part of something shared. Let that connection expand, dissolving any feeling of isolation. You are not alone. You are in relationship—with others, with the world, with what matters most.

Creativity: Recall a moment of creative inspiration—when an idea sparked, a solution revealed itself or you felt fully immersed in artistic expression. Creativity is limitless, flowing, alive. Open yourself to that energy now, allowing fresh insights and possibilities to emerge effortlessly.

Take a few deep breaths, letting these qualities settle within you. They are not fleeting states—you can return to them at any time. Carry this presence with you, knowing that your Self-energy is always available, always waiting to guide you.

Chairwork Dialogue

This exercise helps create space between Self and a part by physically shifting perspectives. It also gives you the opportunity to access a part more directly, by sitting in its seat and allowing it to speak for itself. Sometimes it's surprising what a part shares when given a voice in this way. Rather than thinking *about* the part, you get to speak *from* it—and that shift can offer powerful insight and connection.

Set up two chairs facing each other in a quiet space. One represents your Self, and the other represents the part you wish to engage with. You will move between the two seats as you embody each perspective. If you prefer, you can also use objects like dolls, action figures, pillows or stuffed animals to represent your Self and the part.

Sit in one chair as Self. Take a few deep breaths, grounding yourself in curiosity and openness.

Imagine the part you want to communicate with sitting in the opposite chair. Notice what emotions or sensations arise as you focus on it.

From the Self chair, speak directly to the part, expressing curiosity about its role and needs. You might ask:
- What are you feeling right now?
- What are you trying to protect me from or accomplish for me?
- When did you first take on this role?
- What do you need from me?

Move to the other chair and embody the part. Respond as if you are the part, expressing its emotions and beliefs as honestly as possible.

Continue switching chairs as needed, allowing a natural dialogue to unfold. Stay open to what the part wants to share, even if it feels resistant.

When the conversation feels complete, return to the Self chair and take a few deep breaths, integrating what you've learned.

Journaling from Self

This exercise helps you strengthen the voice of Self by tapping into its clarity and wisdom through writing.

Find a quiet space and connect with your Self-energy. Close your eyes and settle into your body. If any parts feel active—worrying, planning or criticizing—gently let them know they can step back for now. Connect with the qualities of calm, curiosity and clarity. If it helps, recall a moment when you felt deeply grounded or at peace.

Bring to mind a challenge, question or issue you're currently facing.

Begin writing from Self. Once you pick a topic or question, allow the words to flow as if your Self were speaking directly to you. Trust whatever comes. Let the wisdom of Self emerge naturally, without judgment or overthinking.

If a part interrupts, acknowledge it with care. You can briefly note its concerns, then return to writing from Self's perspective.

When you feel complete, reread what you've written. Let the words of your Self fully land.

Journaling from a Part

This exercise helps you connect with a part by giving it a direct voice on the page. Often, parts carry emotions, beliefs and memories that remain unspoken or dismissed. By allowing a part to express itself freely, without judgment or interruption, you can gain deeper insight into its role, concerns and needs.

Identify a part that has been activated recently. Take a few grounding breaths, letting it know you're here to listen.

Begin writing from the part's perspective. Let it speak in its own words, expressing its emotions, history and concerns without censoring or filtering.

Allow the part to explore its role. What does it believe its job is? How does it try to help or protect you? What fears or desires drive it?

What hurts or burdens is this part holding? Does it carry pain from the past, unresolved grief, shame or the weight of unrealistic expectations? Let it express what it's been holding onto and how that has impacted it.

Ask what the part most needs from you. Does it want reassurance, acknowledgment, relief or a change in how it's being treated? Write down whatever arises.

When you feel complete, shift back into Self-energy. Take a few breaths, then reread what you've written from a place of curiosity and compassion. Notice any new understanding that emerges.

Δ

When we are in Self, we are no longer trapped inside our parts' fears, agendas, pain or urgency. We can hold them without becoming them. We can hear their stories without losing ourselves in them. Self creates space for our parts to step forward—not to take over, but to be seen and known. The more we connect with Self, the more we see that we are not just the sum of our fears, wounds and strategies. It is through Self that we find true belonging. Our parts can experience connection and acceptance here, because Self is an inner sanctuary. It is stable, clear and unshaken by the noise of our inner world—and just as importantly, by the chaos of the outer world. Self allows us to move through life without being consumed by its static, to respond instead of react. And when we learn to lead from this place, we don't have to be at war with ourselves. We can finally come home.

CHAPTER 5
BECOMING SELF-CENTERED IN BODY, HEART AND MIND

By now, we've introduced you to a variety of practices designed to help you better access Self-energy. These tools have laid the groundwork for a deeper connection with Self and an increased capacity to unblend from your parts. However, because accessing Self-energy is so essential to transforming the Shame Triangle—and because it's something many people struggle with—we are devoting another chapter to it.

One of the biggest obstacles to connecting with Self is that Self can sometimes feel too abstract. While the IFS model never intended for Self to be perceived as a detached or mystical entity, it's easy to fall into the trap of viewing it that way. Some of us may imagine Self as a distant observer, hovering above daily experiences, or as a wise but separate presence that subtly influences our parts without fully being part of our lived experience. Similarly, the term "Self-energy" can feel elusive or confusing, leaving people questioning whether they are truly accessing it or just imagining it.

To make Self more tangible, people often rely on metaphors. We compare Self to the conductor of an orchestra or the driver of a car, emphasizing its role in harmonizing and guiding our inner system. Others look to concepts like Buddha-nature, the soul or the higher self, which offer a spiritual or philosophical lens for understanding it. While these metaphors can be helpful (and we appreciate them and use them throughout the book), they also pose a challenge: They define Self by pointing outward to something else, rather than anchoring it in our direct experience. This definition can unintentionally make Self seem like something separate from us, rather than a natural and embodied presence within us.

Another challenge people often face is that even when they understand Self, they may not have the foundational skills necessary for parts work. While some people can easily access Self and/or engage with their parts, others may find themselves too blended, too overwhelmed or too locked in the belief patterns of parts to work with their parts effectively. For many, attempting parts work without the necessary inner stability can lead to becoming flooded with emotions, getting stuck in loops of self-criticism or even experiencing trauma-related flashbacks. This is not a personal failure or even a sign that parts work isn't for you—it simply means that you need to develop certain core capacities first. And this makes sense—most of us were never taught how to be with our emotions, relate to our inner world or tend to ourselves with compassion. Of course it can feel difficult, especially when we're trying to do it alone, without the support of a therapist, coach or guide.

Through our practices with clients, we've observed that successful parts work often requires three key foundational skills:
- **Regulating the nervous system** when it becomes dysregulated, creating a sense of safety in the body.
- **Connecting to and speaking from emotions**, identifying feelings and needs without becoming overwhelmed.

- **Recognizing thought patterns and beliefs** that shape the mind, while understanding that these constructs may not always be true or helpful.

When people struggle with parts work, it's often because they haven't yet fully developed one or more of these skills. For example, someone may have strong emotional awareness and be able to name their feelings, but lack the ability to calm themselves when dysregulated, which makes it difficult to stay present with their feelings. Another person may be highly attuned to their bodily sensations but have rigid thought patterns that keep them stuck in self-judgment. These gaps can make accessing Self and working with parts feel overwhelming, inaccessible or even impossible.

This is especially true when we're trying to do this work alone. Self has the power to regulate the nervous system. When you're connected to Self, your breath slows, your body softens and your whole system begins to settle. For some people, this shift happens easily, especially when you're supported by a practitioner who is anchored in their own Self and helping you stay unblended from your parts. But when we're alone and caught in parts that are afraid, angry or overwhelmed, that shift can be much harder to find. For many of us, struggling to access Self is not due to a lack of effort. If we grew up without consistent coregulation, or if trauma shaped our early experiences, we may not yet have the inner scaffolding that makes a quick pivot into Self-regulation feel possible. This isn't a failure. It's a developmental reality, and it's something we can learn to create for ourselves.

To address both the abstract nature of Self and the need for foundational parts work skills, we created the Self-centered model: a model that makes Self more tangible and accessible by grounding it in the lived experience of the body, heart and mind. Instead of seeing Self as something remote or idealized, this model reveals how Self moves through us—how we feel, express and embody it. Yes, you read "Self-centered" correctly—we're reclaiming *another* so-called negative term. Earlier, we reframed "love triangle" into the Self-Love Triangle, and now, we're taking back "self-centered." For too long, "self-centered" has been an insult—a way to describe someone as selfish, disconnected or focused only on their own needs at the expense of others. But what if being self-centered is actually a good thing?

In the Self-centered model, we redefine Self-centeredness as a state of inner alignment. When we are truly Self-centered, our body, heart and mind function in harmony. This is not selfishness—it is Self-leadership. A person centered in Self is grounded in their body, open in their heart and clear in their mind. From this place, they naturally show up with less self-absorption and more compassion, confidence and connection—not because they are trying to be good, but because they are fully in their center. To be Self-centered is to live from the deepest, truest part of yourself, allowing that energy to guide your actions, emotions and thoughts. When you are Self-centered in the best way, you are both deeply attuned to yourself and fully present with others. It's time to reclaim Self-centeredness—not as a flaw, but as a path to wholeness.

The Self-Centered Model

At the core of the Self-centered model is the understanding that Self is an integrated presence that moves within and through the body, heart and mind—the three interconnected centers of our being. We will explore each center in more detail below, but briefly, each center has its own intelligence and unique role:
- **The body**: Communicates through sensations, guiding us toward safety and grounding. It helps regulate our nervous system and keeps us anchored in the present.
- **The heart**: Serves as our emotional center, where we connect with feelings, needs and relational experiences.

It fosters authenticity in our interactions with ourselves and others.
- **The mind**: Functions as the cognitive center, shaping our understanding of reality through thought patterns and beliefs. It helps us discern between helpful perspectives and unhelpful narratives.

Each of our centers carries its own unique gifts and challenges. When they are in balance, we move through life with ease, often without even noticing their support. But when challenges arise, they demand our attention, pulling us toward imbalance and disrupting our sense of stability. Challenges and disruptions can happen for many reasons—illness, trauma, chronic stress, genetic predispositions or external pressures—all of which can throw one center off balance, creating a ripple effect that strains the entire system. Without Self-leadership, the body, heart and mind often swing between extremes—overactivity and underactivity, excess and deficiency—creating dissonance, rather than harmony. Because these centers constantly influence one another, imbalance in one can strain the others, just as alignment in one can help bring the rest back into balance. When one of our centers falls out of balance, it tends to show up in specific ways. When Self is not present or available:
- **The body** may become overstimulated (chronic tension, hypervigilance) or shut down (numbness, fatigue).
- **The heart** may become overwhelmed with intense emotions (fear, sadness, anger) or detach from emotion entirely (disconnection, numbness).
- **The mind** may become trapped in racing thoughts and self-criticism, or it may disengage, making it difficult to focus or gain perspective.

With Self online, we can be present with our experience, rather than becoming consumed by it. The body responds rather than reacts, emotions flow without taking over, and thoughts help us rather than control us. Instead of feeling swallowed by pain, stress or overthinking, we can meet each experience from a steadier place. The body's signals become something we listen to, not fear. Emotions are felt, not avoided. Thoughts are noticed, not believed without question. This is the power of being Self-led.

By tuning into these three centers, we can recognize when we are leaning too heavily into one at the expense of the others. Self-leadership does not mean eliminating life's challenges—some difficulties may always remain part of our experience—but it does help us navigate them with greater ease, skill and grace.

Through becoming Self-centered, Self-leadership is both the goal—how we want to show up in the world—and the path we take to get there. Engaging with our body, heart and mind moves us away from disconnection and toward a more present, grounded way of being. This model helps us see where growth is needed at each center, allowing us to recognize what requires attention and care. The process is reciprocal—the more we access Self, the more our centers come into balance, and the more we strengthen these centers, the easier it becomes to lead from Self. By noticing where we need support, we build the awareness and skills to guide our lives not from fear, reactivity or old wounds, but from the clarity and fortitude of Self.

This model also deepens how we engage with parts work in IFS by offering a fuller view of how parts show up in our system. Just as we experience Self through the body, heart and mind, we experience our parts through these centers, too. Whether protective, wounded or managerial, each part expresses itself across our centers. A part may show up physically as tension in the body—a clenched jaw, a tight chest or restless energy. Emotionally, it may carry fear, sadness, anger or longing. Mentally, it may operate through repetitive thoughts or limiting beliefs. By working with parts in this way, we gain a fuller, more nuanced understanding of them, allowing us to see how they manifest across our centers and relate to our entire system. To better your understanding of the centers, the following sections will examine the wisdom of the body, heart and mind: how they guide us, where they get stuck and how we can cultivate a Self-led balance within each one.

The Body Center

As the starting point of our human journey, the body center comes first in being Self-centered. The body is our first home, the foundation of our being. It anchors us in the present, shaping our earliest experiences and serving as our primary interface with the world. Before we have words for our thoughts, before we are conscious of our feelings, we live through sensation, warmth, tension, movement and touch. Long before we understand the world, our body is teaching us how to navigate it. The rush of excitement, the sting of pain, the comfort of an embrace—these early experiences shape the way we relate to everything.

Our body is both our first teacher and the opening chapter of our story. It shows us the sheer joy of being alive: the thrill of running barefoot, the sun's heat on our skin, laughter shaking through our belly, the safety of being held. But just as powerfully, it teaches us through discomfort: a burn that makes us pull away, a loud noise that jolts us, discomfort in our belly alerting us to hunger. These signals come before thought. The nervous system is constantly tuning in, shifting between ease and alertness, drawing us toward safety and away from threat. This is the body's wisdom: an intelligence that doesn't judge, doesn't analyze, just knows. It knows when we feel good, when we don't and what we need to come back to balance. Through sensation, it speaks to us. There's no right or wrong, just the simple truth of how we are in this moment.

When the Body Is Not Self-Centered

When we're not Self-led, our relationship with our body can feel strained, confusing or even beyond our control. Instead of feeling at home in our own skin, we may struggle to understand what our body is telling us—it can feel like we're at odds with our own physiology. Rather than seeing our body as an ally with its own wisdom, we override its instincts and misread its signals or stop hearing them altogether. Industrialization has widened this disconnect by encouraging us to see the body as a machine—something to be optimized, controlled or ignored in the name of productivity. But the body isn't a machine; it's a living system that relies on sensation to regulate itself. When we lose touch with internal signals—hunger, exhaustion, pain, tension, feelings—our nervous system loses its natural feedback loop. Normally, these signals guide us to rest when we're tired, move when we're restless or seek comfort when we're distressed. But when we disconnect from them, we also lose access to the body's built-in ways of restoring balance.

As a result, stress lingers in the system unchecked. We may live in a constant state of hyperarousal—tense, reactive, on edge—or in hypoarousal, feeling numb, exhausted or shut down. Without awareness of these shifts, we can't respond in ways that bring us back into balance. Over time, being imbalanced weakens our ability to handle life's challenges. Instead of moving through stress and recovering, we feel unease in our bodies, losing an inner sense of safety and well-being.

Society reinforces this disconnect by prioritizing thinking over feeling, logic over intuition, and productivity over rest. From a young age, we're conditioned to push past exhaustion, override hunger and dismiss the need for movement or connection. Meanwhile, health and beauty culture trains us to see our bodies as objects to be modified, controlled or perfected rather than as dynamic, in flux and benefiting from attunement. Instead of listening with curiosity and care, we judge our worth based on external standards like size, fitness or attractiveness. The body becomes something to manage rather than something to inhabit and trust.

This disconnection from the body allows the Shame Triangle to thrive. When we lose touch with our body's signals, we stop responding to its needs and instead try to manage or override them. Rather than listening inward, we look outward, searching for rules or strategies to tell us how to feel, move or exist in our bodies. The Inner Critic then turns the body into a battleground. It picks apart our appearance—our weight, posture, skin, the way we move. It criticizes our energy levels, our hunger cues, our bodily functions. It tells us we are too much or not enough, reinforcing a constant sense that we should be different than we are. It turns natural physical experiences into flaws, making us feel broken for needing rest, for feeling fatigued, for carrying pain. Even normal fluctuations in weight, digestion, hormones or sensory sensitivities become triggers for self-judgment, convincing us that our body is failing us or that we are failing our body.

In an environment of constant criticism, Shame doesn't just arise—it embeds itself in the body. It not only feels bad about the body, but it physically reshapes itself around the criticism through shrinking, hiding or contorting in response. It absorbs the Inner Critic's voice, carrying the weight of its judgments, both physically and emotionally. It pulls inward, tensing muscles, rounding shoulders, trying to disappear.

The Escaper then steps in, trying to escape this discomfort through numbing or control. It drives us toward compulsive attempts to perfect or erase the body—through restrictive dieting, excessive exercise, cosmetic procedures—or into complete disconnection through dissociation, binging or self-harm. Some people over-monitor the body—tracking food, weight or appearance—while feeling increasingly disconnected from how they genuinely feel. Others swing the other way by ignoring the body, neglecting its needs and treating it as irrelevant or burdensome.

All of this creates a body that feels unsafe—a place we are either trapped in or desperately trying to escape. Some of us live in the constant unease of an overactivated nervous system, while others feel cut off, floating through life unanchored. Either way, when the body doesn't feel safe, healing can become much harder to access. Restoring a felt sense of safety in the body supports our ability to tune in—to listen, to stay, to feel—with both Self and the parts that need our attention. At the same time, we can also begin working with the parts of us that carry fear, shame or pain around being in a body, gently helping them see that it may be safer now than it was before.

When the Body Is Self-Centered

When the body center is anchored in Self, we live inside our body rather than hovering above it or disconnecting from it. We experience life through our senses rather than analyzing or controlling our body from a distance. Instead of seeing the body as just a vehicle to transport us through life or a tool in service of the heart and mind, we honor it as a source of wisdom. Self-leadership allows us to listen to and trust our body's cues rather than override or ignore them, guiding us toward what we need to be nourished, balanced and well.

With Self in the lead, we are more attuned to our body's natural rhythms and signals. We notice when we're hungry and what kinds of foods feel supportive, rather than eating out of habit, stress, restriction or just because it's "time to eat." When we move, it's not just for exercise or to hit a step count—it's because our body wants to stretch, sweat, release tension or feel strong. We sense when we need stillness, connection, water, touch or fresh air. We also experience instinctual desires, like sexuality, play, laughter and expression, as natural rhythms to allow and engage with consciously. The more we trust our body, the more it becomes a home to inhabit rather than something to manage or escape from.

A Self-led body center also allows us to meet physical limitations—whether due to aging, illness or ability—with greater acceptance and care. When our body changes, struggles or slows down, Self helps us navigate these realities without shame or resistance. Instead of seeing aging or physical limitations as failures, we can approach them with curiosity and compassion, adapting to what our body needs rather than fighting against it.

Rather than measuring our worth by what our body can do, we learn to be in relationship with it as it is.

When the body is Self-led, it provides a steady foundation for transforming the Shame Triangle into the Self-Love Triangle (chapter 6 gets into this transformation process). With Self in the lead, the Inner Critic shifts from attacking the body to supporting it, becoming an Inner Coach. Instead of berating us for how we look, feel or move, it helps us accept whatever is happening in our body as natural, without judgment. If something needs attention, the Inner Coach guides us toward solutions in a way that is encouraging, rather than paralyzing. It doesn't push us to ignore pain or discomfort, nor does it catastrophize. Instead, it might say, *Your body is asking for rest—let's honor that,* or *This pain is telling you something—let's find a way to care for it.* It reminds us that health is not perfection, strength is not force and worth is not conditional on appearance.

When the Inner Critic becomes an Inner Coach, Shame no longer has the same fuel to feed on. It begins to shift too, no longer shaping our experience of the body through the lens of judgment and fear. Shame no longer carries the same problem-saturated stories. It no longer insists that discomfort means something is wrong with us or that pleasure is undeserved. With Self's support, we can be with whatever raw experience arises in the body—whether it's pain, tension, fatigue or pleasure—without collapsing into a shame story.

The Escapers become Inner Nurturers, learning to turn toward the body rather than away. Instead of numbing, dissociating or pushing through, they help us slow down and tune in. When distress arises, they don't run—they offer comfort, grounding and self-care. If we tend to dissociate, we feel the moment we start drifting away and bring ourselves back into sensation—into the feeling of our feet on the ground, the warmth of our hands, the expansion of our breath. If we have an impulsive Escaper that leaps toward substances or distractions, we notice the urgency in the body first, allowing us to pause before reacting. For overfunctioning Escapers that push us past exhaustion into overwork or constant busyness, we recognize the stress building in the body and learn to release it in ways that restore balance rather than drive us deeper into burnout. With Self in the lead, we sense what our body is holding, where it needs release and how to bring ourselves back to regulation. Instead of being trapped in old patterns, we experience our body as a home—a place we can return to, listen to and trust.

The Heart Center

The heart is the bridge between body and mind—the place where the raw physical sensations of the body meet the stories we tell ourselves in the mind. It's here that empathy, love and genuine emotional connection exist. Feelings are the language of the heart, signaling what we need to stay in harmony with ourselves and others. When we feel warmth or joy, we know our deeper longings are being met. When we sense anxiety or hurt, the heart is alerting us that something essential, like trust, presence or reassurance, is missing.

A Self-led heart welcomes the full spectrum of human emotion. This doesn't mean we eliminate discomfort or pain; rather, we learn to hold our feelings and needs with curiosity and tenderness. The more we stay in touch with the heart, the more we unlock our innate capacity for authenticity, where we can be fully present with our innermost experiences, even when they're vulnerable or messy. Instead of viewing certain emotions as "weak" or "inconvenient," we treat them as important signals guiding us toward deeper connection and emotional honesty. When we tap into the heart's wisdom in this way, something beautiful emerges: the qualities of courage that allow us to see beyond our fears and judgments, compassion that softens the edges of our pain, and empathy that bridges the distance between ourselves and others.

When the Heart Is Not Self-Centered

The heart center faces two main pitfalls when Self-leadership is absent: It either becomes overactive or shuts down. In an overactive state, people feel so swept up in powerful emotions that they lose perspective. A simple disagreement might spiral into a flood of anger or sadness that eclipses everything else, leaving no room to pause and reflect. Rather than seeing their emotions as one part of their experience, they become those emotions, entirely losing any sense of proportion or grounding. While this intensity can reveal deep passion or sensitivity, it also breeds reactivity, moodiness and the sense of being stuck in a perpetual emotional storm.

On the other hand, many people learn to inhibit or disconnect from the heart center altogether. Conditioned by cultural messages that label emotional needs as clingy or dramatic, they may dismiss or bury their feelings before they even fully surface. Over time, this numbness or detachment dulls their awareness of fundamental needs such as closeness, reassurance or joy. Fearing judgment for having "too many feelings," they may pretend not to have them at all—though the heart still registers a quiet ache, longing for expression and validation.

Because emotions can feel overwhelming or uncertain, it's easy to swing between these two extremes—either letting them take over without grounding or shutting them down completely. In both cases, we risk confusing genuine emotional truth with mental interpretations. This confusion often shows up when couples try to discuss a conflict. Instead of sharing their feelings—sadness, hurt, loneliness—the partners may speak in judgments, thoughts and interpretations of the mind. They may say things like "I feel ignored" or "I feel manipulated." These are not actual emotions, but mental conclusions about the other person's behavior. Instead of expressing their hearts, they're describing what they believe the other person is doing. Statements like "I feel like you don't care" may sound vulnerable, yet often carry an implicit accusation—"You're dismissing me on purpose"—which typically gives rise to defensiveness rather than understanding.

This challenge appears on the receiving end as well. Even when one partner bravely offers genuine feelings—naming their loneliness, hurt or fear—it's often heard as blame. Instead of recognizing that these raw emotions are invitations to empathize and connect, the listener perceives them as an attack. Feeling ashamed or wrongly accused, they might argue, shut down or rationalize their behavior to avoid the discomfort of hearing about someone else's pain. In the process, both partners sidestep the authenticity that could deepen their connection, further undervaluing the heart and over-relying on the mind.

It's also common for people to judge their emotions as irrational, illogical or disproportionate. One part of us might feel something strongly, while another part insists we shouldn't be feeling that way—or that the feeling is too big, too long-lasting or just doesn't match the situation. But more often than not, our emotions *do* make sense when we pause and turn toward the part of us that's feeling this way. Often, it's a part that wasn't allowed to feel in the past, that holds an old wound or that's been triggered by something in the present. What might seem irrational from the mind's perspective often has a clear emotional logic when felt through the heart. When we stop analyzing and start listening, we usually discover there's a very good reason for what we're feeling.

These distortions set the stage for the Shame Triangle to take hold in our emotional lives. The Inner Critic reframes natural longings for closeness or care as character flaws—telling us *I'm too sensitive* or *I'm too needy*. It can also flip the script, condemning us for not feeling enough. In such moments, we may even search online for reasons to label ourselves as narcissistic or otherwise disordered, desperately trying to explain why we "should" have a different emotional response. We also tend to judge ourselves harshly when our emotions don't match an imagined ideal. We might think we're not "sad enough" over a loss or not "happy enough" about a success. Or perhaps we feel two seemingly opposite emotions at once—like deep sorrow and relief after ending a relationship or leaving a job—and the Inner Critic scolds us for failing to pick the "correct" feeling. Yet it's completely normal to experience contradictory emotions about the same situation. The heart is naturally expansive enough to hold multiple truths simultaneously, but the Inner Critic tells us only certain emotions are acceptable, allowed or appropriate. This policing of our inner world amplifies shame and confusion, convincing us that something is wrong with us for having complex feelings that don't fit into a single, tidy label.

Shame then weighs heavily on the heart, embedding a constant undertone of embarrassment and self-doubt: *Something is wrong with me because I feel this way.* Rather than validating what we feel, we assume our emotions are proof of some deeper flaw. Meanwhile, Escapers try to escape these feelings entirely or only focus on the ones that seem safe, acceptable or allowed. Some turn to distractions, addictions or endless busyness to numb the heart's pain and avoid emotions they don't know how to process. Others become fixated on maintaining a "positive mindset" and avoid emotions like sadness, anger or grief altogether, convincing themselves that they should only feel gratitude, peace or happiness. Whether through avoidance or selective attention, these strategies disconnect us from the full wisdom of the heart.

When the Heart Is Self-Centered

A Self-led heart allows us to experience emotions fully but not chaotically. Instead of swinging between emotional overwhelm or detachment, we can be present with what we feel without being overtaken by it. When sadness or anger arises, we acknowledge it: "I feel sad," "I feel angry." This simple act of naming emotions creates space between feeling and reaction, allowing us to relate to our emotions with curiosity and steadiness rather than avoidance or amplification.

Being Self-centered in the heart also helps us recognize that emotions serve a purpose—they signal unmet needs, values or boundaries that require attention. If we feel sadness after a conflict with a friend, it's not a flaw; it's a sign that we value connection and respect in our relationships. Rather than judging ourselves as "too needy" for wanting closeness, we see our feelings as insights rather than problems. We understand them as part of a natural flow—one that offers guidance, rather than chaos.

When the Inner Critic shifts into being an Inner Coach (more in chapter 6), emotions are no longer something to battle against or prove wrong. Instead of questioning whether we should feel a certain way, we recognize that every emotion makes sense in context. The Inner Coach helps us work with our emotions rather than against them, offering perspective without dismissal. If we feel anger, it might remind us that something important to us is being threatened. If we feel sadness, it might encourage us to stay with our feeling of sadness rather than assume it means something is broken. The Inner Coach doesn't rush us past our emotions, but helps us move through them in a way that allows for expression without getting stuck.

Shame no longer distorts our emotions or buries them under self-doubt. We allow the truth of what we feel, even when it's uncomfortable. Instead of assuming emotions need justification or permission, we let them be. The parts of us that turn toward us—whether an Inner Nurturer or Inner Coach—help us see that there's always a good reason we feel the way we do. Rather than labeling our emotions as "too much" or "not enough," we acknowledge that they are part of being human, revealing what matters to us.

With Inner Nurturers in place, emotions don't have to be avoided, exaggerated or controlled. There is space to feel deeply without becoming overwhelmed. Inner Nurturers help us stay present with emotions we once tried to push away, making it easier to sit with grief, disappointment, longing or love without bracing against them. Inner Nurturers provide the warmth that allows us to settle, and the reassurance that reminds us we don't have to go through it alone. They help us recognize when we need comfort and guide us toward what would be most supportive, whether that's connection, movement, stillness or simply letting ourselves feel.

Over time, a Self-centered heart builds emotional resilience. We become more comfortable with vulnerability, trusting that we can hold difficult emotions without being consumed by them. We no longer feel the need to tiptoe around or explode with unprocessed emotions—instead, we integrate them into a broader understanding of ourselves. This integration deepens our authenticity, allowing us to be more present both within ourselves and with others. Recognizing how difficult it can be to sit with vulnerable feelings, we become more empathetic, creating safer emotional spaces for others as well.

A Self-led heart also allows us to connect more deeply with love. This love is not grasping or dependent—it is an open presence that flows from within rather than something we must chase externally. We no longer love from a place of fear or lack, but with expansiveness, warmth and the ability to hold both closeness and freedom. Love stops being something we cling to or control and instead becomes something we embody.

The Mind Center

The human mind is a marvel of creativity and innovation, often considered the defining feature that sets us apart from other species. Through our unique capacity for language, storytelling, invention and abstract thought, we've built civilizations, formed cultural identities and expanded our understanding of the universe.

You might think of the mind as a four-in-one device: an antenna that picks up signals from the environment, a filter that determines which information matters, a tuner that focuses our attention, and a transmitter that shares our thoughts with others. When guided by Self, this intricate system becomes a source of clarity and vision. We use our mental gifts to solve problems, create art, engage in meaningful dialogue and shape our own futures. In this optimal state, the mind isn't just a chatterbox or a problem generator—it's a wellspring of insight, curiosity and connection that makes life richer and more purposeful.

When the Mind Is Not Self-Centered

Without the balancing presence of Self-leadership, the same abilities that make the mind so powerful can turn chaotic. The antenna picks up an onslaught of intrusive thoughts, worries and external demands. The filter becomes clouded by biases—some inherited from family or culture, others formed through trauma or unmet needs. The tuner either locks onto worst-case scenarios, leading to a hyperfocus on doom and gloom, or struggles to find any clear channel at all. And the transmitter, rather than broadcasting wisdom, repeats anxious ruminations, repetitive fears or critical messages.

Instead of serving as a tool for focus, awareness and growth, the mind can become a barrier, denying the heart's emotions and the body's needs. It rationalizes away pain, explains feelings rather than feeling them and pushes through discomfort to maintain control. In these moments, the mind can swing between frantic overthinking and numbing disengagement—lost in spirals of "what ifs" one moment and mentally checked out the next. Often driven by fear or shame, it leans on cognitive defenses like minimizing, catastrophizing or rationalizing—temporary shields that ultimately keep us disconnected from our bodies and hearts.

Because the mind naturally tells stories, it can easily become trapped in problem-saturated ones. The mind is built to find patterns and make sense of things, but without Self-leadership, it latches onto the wrong conclusions—especially about ourselves. Enter the Inner Critic, who fills the mind with harsh, looping thoughts—self-judgment, impossible standards and a constant search for flaws. It dissects every mistake, replays past failures and keeps a running tally of where we fall short. Shame settles in by making these thoughts feel definitive, even when they're just one narrow interpretation. Instead of seeing them as opinions or learned beliefs, we accept them as facts about who we are. The mind tightens around these judgments, leaving little room to question them.

Meanwhile, Escapers try to flee the weight of these thoughts, either by tuning out or by staying stuck in thinking itself. Some try to leave the mind entirely, while others double down, convinced that if we just analyze more, plan better or figure everything out, we can avoid discomfort. In both cases, they treat the mind as either something to escape or something to overrely on, but this strategy only creates more mental noise, leaving us further disconnected from Self.

When the Mind Is Self-Centered

When the mind is Self-led, its energy becomes clear and constructive. We're no longer caught in a battle with our thoughts—we're in relationship with them. Rather than controlling, fixing or avoiding them, we meet them with interest and spaciousness. Imagine standing at the edge of a rushing river. When parts are in control, you're caught in the current, swept away by whatever thought or worry is strongest. You tumble through doubts, fears and endless loops of analysis. But with Self in the lead, you step onto the riverbank. The river still flows, but you're no longer submerged in it. From this grounded place, thoughts become things we can observe, explore and respond to rather than things that dictate our experience.

A Self-centered mind is spacious and reflective. It can hold multiple perspectives at once without getting lost in them. It welcomes complexity without spiraling into confusion. Instead of scrambling for certainty, it remains open to possibilities. Mental activity serves a purpose rather than running unchecked. We can think critically, solve problems and engage in deep reflection without being consumed by overthinking. The mind becomes a tool for insight rather than a battleground for anxious, ruminative loops.

Even when we live with ongoing cognitive differences or mental health conditions—like neurodivergence, anxiety, depression or learning challenges—Self-leadership allows us to relate to them differently. Rather than trying to eliminate or override these experiences, we begin to recognize them as part of our unique cognitive landscape. From this perspective, we can approach them with more understanding and less shame. These experiences may shape how we move differently through the world, but they can also carry their own gifts of sensitivity, insight, depth, intuition, creativity, pattern recognition or out-of-the-box thinking. A Self-led mind helps us see the whole picture, honoring both the challenges and the strengths we hold and making space for how our minds are uniquely wired to engage with life.

Self-leadership also transforms how the Inner Critic, Shame and Escapers operate. When guided by Self, these parts shift into the Self-Love Triangle, creating a mental environment that fosters curiosity, encouragement and thoughtful exploration. The Inner Critic becomes an Inner Coach, offering guidance rather than tearing us down. Instead of dwelling on flaws or reinforcing rigid standards, it helps us think constructively. It might ask, *What would help me learn from this mistake?* or *How can I approach this challenge in a way that supports me?* Rather than fixating on shortcomings, it points to our values, highlights what truly matters and keeps us focused on solutions.

Shame no longer clings to stories of failure or deficiency. With Self's support, it allows us to see difficult thoughts as passing mental states rather than absolute truths. Instead of feeling trapped in judgment, we can acknowledge when an old belief surfaces and recognize it for what it is—just a thought, not a definition of who we are. This shift makes space for a more honest and supportive relationship with ourselves.

Escapers become Inner Nurturers, no longer running from discomfort but helping us engage with our thoughts in a way that feels safe. They don't try to escape the mind or control it—they help us care for it. They encourage us to take mental breaks when needed, step away when we're overwhelmed and return with fresh perspective. They remind us that clarity comes not from overthinking but from allowing space for insight to emerge.

When the mind is centered in Self, thoughts are no longer something to fear or control. We develop trust in our ability to witness them, engage with them and, when necessary, let them go. There is less noise, less urgency and less grasping for certainty. Instead of being consumed by our thinking, we use it as a resource—one that supports growth, creativity and deeper understanding.

Evaluating Your Three Centers

This self-evaluation is designed to help you identify where you may experience excess (overactivity) or deficiency (underactivity) within your body, heart and mind centers. Read through the questions in each section, marking statements that apply to you and reviewing the recommendations to bring greater Self-leadership into that area.

The Body Center: Sensation, Safety and Regulation

Signs of Excess (Overactivity)
- ☐ I frequently feel restless, tense or hypervigilant.
- ☐ I struggle to sit still and find relaxation difficult.
- ☐ I experience chronic pain, headaches or physical stress symptoms.
- ☐ I react impulsively or physically when stressed (e.g., pacing, fidgeting, clenching).

☐ I overuse physical stimulation (e.g., excessive exercise, thrill-seeking, substance use).

Self-Centered Adjustments
- **Slow down movement:** Instead of intense exercise, try restorative practices like slow stretching, yin yoga or floating in water.
- **Soothing sensory input:** Engage in self-massage, weighted blankets, warm baths or soft textures to signal safety to the nervous system.
- **Progressive relaxation:** Systematically tense and release muscles to help your body register the difference between tension and ease.
- **Nervous system discharge:** Engage in shaking, dancing or stomping to help release excess stored energy.
- **Nature recalibration:** Spend time in grounding natural settings (gardens, forests, near water) to settle overstimulation.

Signs of Deficiency (Underactivity)
☐ I feel numb, disconnected or dissociated from my body.
☐ I often forget to eat, hydrate or rest.
☐ My breath is shallow or restricted, and I rarely notice it.
☐ I struggle to sense physical cues like hunger, fatigue or discomfort.
☐ I avoid movement or physical activity, feeling lethargic or withdrawn.

Self-Centered Adjustments
- **Reawaken sensation:** Use temperature contrast (warm/cool), textured objects or movement like rolling a ball under your feet to gently engage the body.
- **Re-engage the breath:** Try active breathwork to bring energy into the body.

- **Move in micro-ways:** Start small—stretch your fingers, roll your shoulders, sway side to side—rather than forcing intense exercise.
- **Reestablish rhythm:** Drumming, rhythmic walking or gentle bouncing can help synchronize internal awareness with external movement.
- **Reconnect through touch:** Place your hands on different body parts and offer a simple acknowledgment: "I am here."

The Heart Center: Emotional Awareness and Connection

Signs of Excess (Overactivity)
- ☐ I feel emotionally flooded or overwhelmed by my feelings.
- ☐ I take on others' emotions as my own and struggle with boundaries.
- ☐ I frequently feel intense emotional highs and lows.
- ☐ I become reactive, defensive or easily triggered in relationships.
- ☐ I struggle to contain my emotions and often vent without feeling relief.

Self-Centered Adjustments
- **Create space and containment for emotions:** Imagine placing your feelings in or on to something tangible—a journal, a box, even a mental shelf—so you can notice what you're feeling without getting pulled under.
- **Hold boundaries with care:** Remind yourself, "I can be present without taking this on." You can respond to messages and emails at your own pace. In conversations, try saying, "I hear you, and I also need a moment to check in with myself."
- **Be specific when naming emotions:** Instead of saying, "I feel awful," try naming what's underneath: "I feel sad

and frustrated." This helps your system process emotions more clearly.
- **Reduce emotional input when needed:** If you're feeling overloaded, step back from news, social media or emotionally intense interactions. Protecting your capacity is part of staying Self-centered.
- **Use grounding touch:** A hand on your chest or arms crossed over your body can signal safety to your nervous system. You might say, "It's safe to feel. I can stay with myself through this."

Signs of Deficiency (Underactivity)
- ☐ I feel emotionally disconnected or detached from my feelings.
- ☐ I have trouble identifying what I'm feeling beyond basic emotions like "fine" or "tired."
- ☐ I suppress emotions, avoiding vulnerability or deeper connections.
- ☐ I struggle to express my needs or desires in relationships.
- ☐ I feel numb, unmotivated or isolated in social settings.

Self-Centered Adjustments
- **Name even subtle emotions:** If big feelings feel inaccessible, start with small shifts: "Do I feel neutral? Slightly unsettled? A little lighter?"
- **Use music or art to evoke feeling:** Listen to songs that match what you might be feeling underneath. Engage in expressive movement or drawing.
- **Write letters to yourself:** Even if you struggle to verbalize emotions, writing from the heart (to yourself, or to a younger you) can open expression.
- **Reconnect through physical affection:** Allow safe, supportive touch—self-hugs, hand over heart, snuggling a pet—to ease emotional access.

- **Engage in coregulation:** Spend time with a trusted friend or safe, attuned person who naturally helps you feel more open.

The Mind Center: Thought Patterns and Perspective

Signs of Excess (Overactivity)
☐ My thoughts race, and I often overanalyze everything.
☐ I get stuck in self-criticism, rumination or anxious "what if" scenarios.
☐ I intellectualize my emotions instead of feeling them.
☐ I have trouble turning my mind "off" and experience mental exhaustion.
☐ I rely too much on logic, dismissing intuition or emotional insights.

Self-Centered Adjustments
- **Practice "thought watching":** Instead of engaging with thoughts, picture them floating by like clouds in the sky or leaves on a stream.
- **Shift into the body or heart:** When caught in overthinking, ask, "What do I feel in my body?" or "What is my heart saying?"
- **Reframe mental loops:** If a thought keeps repeating, write down three alternative perspectives to soften its grip.
- **Set "worry appointments":** Schedule five minutes of "worry time" daily to acknowledge fears—then redirect your focus afterward.
- **Do something physically engaging:** Handwork (gardening, crafting, playing an instrument) helps shift you from the mind into embodied presence.

Signs of Deficiency (Underactivity)
☐ I have difficulty focusing, and my mind often feels foggy or sluggish.

☐ I avoid self-reflection, preferring distraction over introspection.
☐ I struggle to make decisions and frequently feel indecisive.
☐ I have trouble forming clear thoughts or articulating my experiences.
☐ I feel disconnected from my own perspective and rely on others to define my reality.

Self-Centered Adjustments
- **Ask grounding questions:** What do I know for sure in this moment? What is one thought I want to claim today?
- **Use structured thinking tools:** Write down pros/cons, lists or mind maps to engage clarity.
- **Verbally process thoughts:** Speak aloud (even to yourself) to help organize mental space.
- **Read or listen to engaging material:** Expose your mind to thought-provoking books, podcasts or discussions to reawaken curiosity.
- **Move with intention:** Walking while thinking (or talking to yourself out loud) helps reconnect mental clarity with movement.

Integration and Reflection: Bringing the Three Centers into Balance

Look at your responses across all three centers.
- Which center(s) had the most excess?
- Which center(s) had the most deficiency?
- Which center needs the most care? What is one small action you can take today to bring more balance to that center?
- Which center do you feel most Self-centered in—where you most often feel aligned, grounded and resourced? How can you draw on the strengths of that center to support the others?

- What does Self-leadership feel like for you? How do you know when you're leading from Self rather than from a center's excess or deficiency?

Δ

Being Self-centered is not something you master and complete—it's a practice of returning to yourself, again and again. Some days, you will feel steady and centered. Other days, Self may feel out of reach. This is part of being human. What matters isn't always staying in Self, but knowing how to find your way back. Every time you listen to your body, allow an emotion or question a thought, you are strengthening your ability to lead from Self. This work is also not about becoming perfect—it's about becoming present. It's about knowing that you can meet yourself exactly as you are, with all your contradictions, struggles and strengths. It's about making space inside yourself to hold it all. Even when Self feels distant, it hasn't disappeared. It is always here, beneath the surface, waiting for you to turn toward it.

So rather than asking yourself whether you're getting this "right," ask yourself some simpler questions:

- How can I inhabit my body with more presence?
- How can I allow my emotions with care and authenticity?
- How can I meet my thoughts with curiosity and discernment?

CHAPTER 6
DIALOGUING WITH YOUR PARTS

Now that you have developed more capacity and skills in being Self-centered, we can begin the journey of directly engaging in dialogue with your Shame Triangle parts. From this state of Self-energy, the Shame Triangle can transform into the Self-Love Triangle, where each part is freed from its former role. The Inner Critic, once harsh and demeaning, evolves into an Inner Coach—one that encourages us, holds us to healthy standards and provides guidance rather than punishment. The Escapers, which previously turned away from pain and difficult emotions, become Inner Nurturers—turning toward us in moments of struggle to help us regulate, self-soothe and stay present as emotions rise and fall.

Interestingly, even though people often have multiple Escaper parts, these parts commonly converge into a single Inner Nurturer, rather than each Escaper transforming separately. As you move through this process, you may discover that one or several Nurturers arise. There's no right result—what matters is what your system needs and how care and support naturally form within you.

Shame, however, doesn't simply become a different part. Rather than turning into something new, it dissolves into what was always there: our Raw Experience. It's our unfiltered encounter with the full spectrum of our emotions—the grief, the joy, the fear, the longing, the rage, the tenderness—before any part steps in to reduce, judge or reshape them. When we were coming up with what to call the product of Shame's transformation, we initially considered naming it Vulnerability or Tenderness. These names captured part of the truth, but they didn't include the full experience—the moments of hopelessness, anger or helplessness, and the emotions that don't feel soft or tender. Shame also isn't only a reaction to challenging feelings; it can just as easily arise in response to joy, confidence, desire or pleasure. Many of us learned—directly or indirectly—that feeling too much, whether painful or pleasurable, was unacceptable. Over time, we internalized the belief that certain emotions were dangerous, that something about us was wrong for experiencing them.

Shame has always been a reaction to emotions we didn't know how to have. As children, we didn't yet have the capacity to hold these experiences on our own, and the adults around us often didn't know how to help us. Whether through direct messages or subtle cues, we were taught that these feelings were wrong—that they should be hidden, controlled or avoided. Left without the tools to process them, we absorbed the belief that the feelings themselves were the problem. And so, rather than learning how to sit with them, we learned how to escape.

This is why Shame's transformation isn't as flashy as those of the other parts. The Inner Critic becoming an Inner Coach, the Escapers turning into Inner Nurturers—these shifts sound inspiring. But our Raw Experience is not about becoming something else; it is about returning to what was always there. It is about learning to sit with discomfort, to be with what is. It's about reclaiming our ability to feel what we feel—without pushing it away, running from it or believing it means something is wrong with us. It's not just about vulnerability and tenderness, though those are part of it. It's also about staying present with powerlessness, hopelessness, rage, grief and uncertainty—the emotions we are most likely to refuse.

Think about the moments that bring up these feelings the most: witnessing injustice, war or devastation in the world. Facing loss, illness or deep personal hardship. These experiences stir something primal in us. They remind us of how small we can feel, how little control we sometimes have. And when we don't know how to be with these feelings, we often try to escape them—through distraction, denial, numbing or throwing ourselves into action as a way to avoid feeling powerless. But these emotions don't need to be erased or controlled; they need the space to be held.

The Absent but Implicit

Before you can begin *talking* to your parts, you need to make sure you know how to *listen*. One of the biggest challenges people encounter when engaging with their Shame Triangle parts is that these parts speak in absolutes—harsh judgments and black-and-white declarations that leave no room for nuance. Statements like *You're a failure* or *You'll never get it right* don't invite discussion. They position us in a trap where the only available responses seem to be either agreeing (*You're right, I am a failure*) or fighting back (*That's not true! Stop saying that!*). But neither approach leads to a productive conversation with the part. People often give up on talking to their parts because they don't know how to listen for the deeper longings beneath these harsh statements. It's easy to miss that these extreme judgments, as painful as they are, are actually pointing toward something important. Before we engage directly with our parts, we need a new way of listening—one that allows us to hear beyond the words, to what these parts really need.

One way to do this is through the concept of the *absent but implicit*. This idea from narrative therapy helps us recognize what's beneath the surface of our complaints, frustrations or pain—what's not being said, but is still shaping our experience. When we talk about a problem, we tend to focus on what's wrong. For example, if someone says, "I feel unappreciated at work," the explicit message is frustration about being undervalued. But if we listen more closely and ask ourselves what must matter to them for this to hurt, we might see that beneath their complaint is a longing for respect, recognition or feeling like their efforts have meaning. These values are *absent* from the person's words, but they are still present, shaping the person's experience, *implicit* in what they are saying.

We make sense of our experiences through contrast. We often know what we *don't* want because, somewhere inside, we already hold an idea of what we *do* want. If someone says, "No one ever listens to me," their frustration is clear—but what's missing in their words is the longing to be heard and understood. If someone says, "I can never get anything right," the judgment may carry a hidden hope of being competent, capable or valued. Every complaint or criticism carries a shadow of something important—an unspoken desire, a deeply held value, a glimpse of what we wish could be true. If we only listen to what's explicit— the frustration, the hurt, the judgment—we can feel stuck. But when we start listening for what's absent but implicit, we shift. We stop being trapped in the problem and start recognizing what we actually want.

Double Listening: A New Way to Hear Your Parts

One way to uncover the absent but implicit is through a narrative therapy technique called double listening—a way of tuning in beyond the surface of what is said. Instead of taking judgments, complaints or emotional reactions at face value, we "turn the coin over" and ask: What does this reveal about what truly matters to this person? Double listening means paying attention to both the words being spoken and the deeper needs, feelings and values that may not yet have been named. It acknowledges that our emotions and stories are never just one-dimensional; they carry within them unspoken commitments, hopes and deeply held beliefs.

Here are some examples of how double listening helps us uncover the absent but implicit:
- **Anger**: When someone expresses anger, they're not just upset about what happened. Anger often signals a sense of injustice, a need for protection or a desire for fairness. Beneath the anger, there may be an unspoken hope for respect, boundaries or safety.
- **Sadness**: Expressing sadness often means mourning a loss. But implicit in that sadness is something valuable—love, appreciation or connection to what was lost. Sadness reveals what we cherish.
- **Fear**: Fear is usually about anticipating something painful or uncertain. But hidden in fear is an idea of what would feel safe, secure or reassuring.
- **Despair**: Despair can look like the loss of hope, but if we listen closely, we might hear the echoes of past dreams and aspirations—things that once felt possible and meaningful. These hopes can still be reclaimed or reshaped.
- **Hurt**: When someone expresses hurt, it's often because something they value—trust, care or recognition—has been violated. At its core, hurt carries a longing for healing, repair or acknowledgment.

We can also use double listening to reframe judgments and self-perceptions:
- **Injustice**: When people express outrage at injustice, they aren't just angry at what's wrong. Their response reflects values of fairness, dignity and a vision of a just world. Seeing these values can help us turn frustration into purpose.
- **Burdened**: Feeling burdened isn't just about having too much responsibility—it often signals devotion to

something that matters. Some burdens are imposed, but others are chosen out of love or duty. Naming these values can help us shift the weight from resentment to meaning.
- **Woundedness**: Shame often distorts wounds into proof of being broken or unfixable. But double listening reveals that woundedness is tied to ideas of healing, strength and what it means to be whole. These beliefs can guide us toward recovery.
- **Unworthiness**: Judgments of unworthiness manifest as self-doubt or harsh self-judgment, but beneath them is a longing for acceptance, belonging and love. Seeing this longing can help us transform shame into self-compassion.

When we find ourselves stuck in painful emotions or repetitive complaints, we can ask: What does this struggle reveal about what truly matters to me? This kind of inquiry can become a regular practice—one that brings clarity not just to our emotions but to what we value most. And when we recognize what we long for, we can start finding ways to actively bring more of it into our lives.

In the context of transforming the Shame Triangle, the concept of the absent but implicit is especially potent. Our Shame Triangle parts don't speak in direct requests. They typically don't gently ask for reassurance, belonging or safety. Instead, they speak in extremes: *You're disgusting, No one will ever love you, I'll always be this way.* These parts believe they are protecting us, but their language is punishing. If we take these statements at face value, we will either collapse under them or argue against them—neither of which helps. But when we listen for what is absent but implicit, we start hearing the deeper truth:
- **The Inner Critic** speaks in harsh absolutes: *You're gross, You're failing* or *You'll never get it right.* It seems rigid and punishing, but beneath that criticism is something deeply invested in our well-being. The absent but implicit is a desire for security, integrity and alignment with what matters most. The Inner Critic fears failure because it

values success and wants to have worth. It points out flaws because it cares about being loved or doing things well. It holds high standards not to punish us, but because it believes meeting them will keep us safe, accepted or worthy.
- **Shame** weighs us down with messages of inadequacy: *I'm unlovable, I'm broken* or *I don't belong*. On the surface, it seems to insist we are deficient, but beneath that painful narrative is a longing to be included, valued and allowed to be as we are. The absent but implicit is the need to exist freely. Shame is not just about feeling unworthy—it is about yearning for the right to take up space, to be seen and accepted, to know that our inner experience is valid and allowed.
- **The Escaper** urges us to check out, avoid or numb: *I can't handle this, This is too much* or *I just need to get away*. It appears to be fleeing discomfort, but if we listen more closely, we hear a part that feels overwhelmed and underresourced. The absent but implicit is a longing for relief, yes—but also for support, capacity and a sense of agency. The Escaper doesn't avoid because it's careless; it avoids because it hasn't yet learned how to stay present without drowning. Beneath the urge to escape is a deep wish to re-engage—when it finally feels safe enough to do so. It's not apathy. It's a hope for rest, regulation and the ability to face life without burning out.

A Few Common Concerns Before You Begin

Before we jump into dialogue with your parts, we want to pause and name a few common concerns that often come up during this kind of work. Since this isn't a one-size-fits-all process, it's important to acknowledge the real questions and hesitations that can surface along the way.

Which Part Do We Begin Working With?

Different therapeutic models take different approaches to working with parts. In IFS, the typical path is to work with protective parts first before addressing wounded or exiled parts. Other approaches tend to focus on whatever part is most activated in the moment.

In our work with the Shame Triangle, we've found that when the Inner Critic shifts first, the entire Triangle begins to change. Once the Inner Critic stops berating Shame, Shame has room to breathe, heal and just be. When those two parts are no longer locked in struggle, the need for Escapers naturally lessens, and the system starts to rebalance. Because of this, in the next section, we begin by working with the Inner Critic, then Shame, and finally the Escapers.

That said, sometimes it makes sense to start elsewhere. If Shame is your most dominant experience, or if Escapers are causing major disruption, it may be best to work with them first to create stability. Sometimes, you need to start by putting out a fire. And remember that this work is not a one-time conversation with each part. A single dialogue can create powerful insights, but real transformation takes time and repetition. Just like learning a new skill or strengthening a muscle, change happens through repeated practice.

But Don't We Need Our Shame Triangle?

Many people believe they need their Inner Critic, Shame and high-functioning Escapers to keep them in line. The fear is that without these parts constantly pushing, judging or warning them about their flaws, they'll become too much, reckless or selfish, or they'll fail to meet expectations. Some people may even fear that they cannot survive without these parts. If these roles were essential to our survival growing up, it makes sense that letting them go or even changing them could feel terrifying.

However, the opposite is often true. When we transform them, we don't lose life—we gain it.

We understand this concern. But in reality, transforming the Shame Triangle doesn't make people less accountable or ethical—it expands their capacity for both. When we're caught in the Shame Triangle, we generally struggle to take true accountability because we get stuck in cycles of criticism, collapse, defensiveness and avoidance. The Inner Critic attacks, Shame paralyzes and Escapers pull us away from what needs to be faced. Escapers often protect us by numbing, distracting or avoiding—but they also show up through people-pleasing. They may say what others want to hear or offer quick apologies, not from true ownership, but from fear of conflict or rejection. This isn't real accountability—it's a fawn response, a survival strategy. Instead of making meaningful repair, we shut down, deflect responsibility or spiral into self-condemnation.

By contrast, when we shift into the Self-Love Triangle, we gain a deeper capacity for self-reflection and integrity. This new internal environment allows us to acknowledge our mistakes without drowning in them. From this place, we can take responsibility, repair harm and make real changes—not out of fear or self-punishment, but from alignment with our values.

Transforming a part doesn't mean stripping away its strengths. It still gets to keep what works—it just operates differently now. Some parts will truly transform, taking on a new role that is a better version of what they once were. Others won't change their identity entirely but will update how they function. Instead of working from fear, shame or avoidance, they align with Self, using their strengths in a way that genuinely supports us. Parts don't have to disappear. They don't even have to fully change their nature. Some will take on a new job, while others will simply learn to work in a way that serves us, rather than keeping us stuck.

What If a Part Doesn't Want to Become an Updated Version of Itself?

So far in this book, we've been describing the typical transformation of the Shame Triangle: the Inner Critic shifts into an Inner Coach, Shame dissolves into your Raw Experience and Escapers coalesce into an Inner Nurturer. Most of the time, this is exactly what happens. These parts tend to want updated roles that are truly helpful and relevant to your life. But that's not always the case.

Some parts don't want a new job—they want to retire. A harsh Inner Critic may realize it's exhausted and ready to step down. An Escaper might no longer feel the need to keep running. Once their burdens are lifted, some parts transform—becoming light, playful, even childlike. Others may shift into quieter allies or on-call advisors, available when needed but no longer in charge. And some parts, once fully seen and released, may simply dissolve—grateful to no longer be weighed down by the responsibilities they once carried. If this happens, it's completely OK. Healing doesn't have to follow a specific script. In these cases, we can either invite new parts to step in and take on protective roles in a healthier way, or rely more fully on Self to meet our needs rather than assigning the role to another part. What matters most isn't whether a part transforms into a specific role but that your internal system becomes more current, supportive and aligned with Self.

The Transformation Process

As we offer you this process, think of it as a flexible guide rather than a rigid formula. Every person's internal world is unique, and transformation happens in different ways. Give yourself the space to explore, adjust and revisit as needed. As you move through the next sections, you can work with the general pattern of your Shame Triangle or focus on a specific Shame Triangle that plays out in certain areas of your life. If you choose the latter, you can always return to the process again for another version of your Shame Triangle.

We also don't recommend doing all this parts work back-to-back. Think of each conversation with your parts like a therapy session or a meaningful journey—one that benefits from reflection. Give yourself time between dialogues to process, notice shifts and allow the work to settle. Even if you prefer to go through the steps more quickly, at least take a break between conversations with each part. The goal isn't to rush through the process, but to create enough space for real change to take hold.

Transforming the Inner Critic

In chapter 2, you gained a general understanding of how your Inner Critic operates. Now, you will engage in a direct dialogue with this part to understand its history and roles, as well as the positive intentions behind its harsh tactics. The key here is to approach your Inner Critic with curiosity about its origin story and connect with its underlying motivations (the absent but implicit), which often stem from a place of care and protection, even if its methods are misguided. When in dialogue with the Inner Critic, you'll also point out how its current strategies, though well-meaning, are ultimately harmful, rather than helpful. During this conversation, you'll invite the Inner Critic to redefine its role, shifting from a harsh, demeaning voice to one of a supportive inner guide that can firmly yet kindly nudge you toward growth.

If the title "Inner Coach" doesn't quite land for you, feel free to create your own. Your Inner Critic could transform into an Inner Cheerleader, Inner Council, Inner Mentor, Inner Sage or Inner Yoda. It's your call! The key is to find a title and role that feels meaningful to you, and that allow this part to retain its protective and motivating qualities while shedding the harsh, self-critical tactics that hold you back. With an open mind and a spirit of collaboration, you can cocreate a new role for this part that aligns with the ways you genuinely need protection and guidance now.

Self LOVE U Inner Critic Process

This exercise is adapted from our book *Polywise*, where we integrate and give our own spin on the IFS and narrative therapy processes to create the Love U process. We have since updated this process and now call it Self LOVE U. It is meant to be used when you are connecting with a part for the first time. In this first encounter, aim to get to know the Inner Critic and its history, and relate to it in ways that will show it you are an ally and can be trusted. During this first round, your goal is simply to connect with this part and establish—or in some cases, reestablish—a relationship. After you've successfully connected with your Inner Critic, you can use the EASE exercise in the appendix to continue deepening your work with this part. The following chapters will further guide you in unburdening the Inner Critic and supporting its transformation into an Inner Coach.

- **Self** Connect with Self-Energy
- **L** Locate the Inner Critic
- **O** Origin Story
- **V** Validate Its Efforts and Intentions
- **E** Educate
- **U** Update

To get the most out of this practice, you will need to be in a space where you can have privacy and time for reflection. Create an environment where you feel safe and won't be distracted or interrupted.

Self Connect with Self-Energy

Close your eyes and turn inward. Take a few deep breaths, letting each exhale settle you into the present moment. If any parts are active, kindly ask them to step back for now. Allow yourself to sink into Self-energy. Rest here for a few moments, or longer if needed, until you feel centered and ready to begin. Take your time to ensure a solid grounding in your Self energy before moving on to the "Locate" step.

L   Locate the Inner Critic

Once centered and grounded, locate your Inner Critic within your physical or psychological space. Where does it show up? Is it a voice inside your head, a feeling within your body or an external presence around you? If it is already outside of you, ask it to locate itself in front of you to talk.

If you experience the Inner Critic inside your body or mind, invite it to externalize by stepping outside of you. Imagine it taking a form and positioning itself at a comfortable distance in front of you. The externalized Inner Critic may appear as a clear humanlike figure, a younger version of yourself or an abstract form, or you may experience it more through intuition, sound or a felt sense rather than visually.

If the Inner Critic is hesitant to engage or resistant to externalizing, reassure it that you are not trying to get rid of it or punish it. Explain that your intention is simply to connect with and understand it better.

Once it's located externally, re-check that you are still centered in Self. Maintain an open, curious stance toward the Inner Critic. Again, if any other parts jump in, kindly ask them to step aside and assure them that you are in Self, which can handle talking to the Inner Critic.

O   Origin Story

Begin getting to know your Inner Critic by asking about its origin story. How long has this part been with you? What life circumstances created it? When did it first appear? What events or experiences contributed to its development? Ask the part what it believes is important for you to know now.

Remember to listen from Self without reliving the part's experiences. If the part overwhelms you, ask it to slow down or imagine it smaller or farther away from you. If memories arise, you can watch them as if you're there, or you can project them onto a screen or phone to watch from a more comfortable distance.

Once you get a good sense of how and why this part came about, inquire about the Inner Critic's intentions, purpose, role or job underneath its critical strategies. Ask: What does this part want for you? What job or role has it taken on? What does this part stand for and what does it stand against? What is it trying to protect you from? What is its intention for you? What is it trying to achieve? How does it believe it's helping you? If the Inner Critic states its intention negatively by saying what it doesn't want for you or what's it's trying to avoid (such as to keep you from getting hurt or to avoid disapproval), continue to inquire into those motivations until you get to the Inner Critic's positive intention (such as, it wants you to be loved, accepted or safe). Understanding this positive protective intention is essential to transform your relationship with the Inner Critic.

V Validate Its Efforts and Intentions

After getting the Inner Critic's origin story and understanding the role it has played, speak from Self to validate and acknowledge this part for how it came about and why it took its particular form. Acknowledge the Inner Critic for trying to keep you safe. We will address its methods for implementing its intention in a later step. For now, just let it know that you see how it's been protecting you and you appreciate what it's been trying to achieve (even if it hasn't always achieved it well).

Validate the Inner Critic's experiences and the challenges it has endured on your behalf. Given the circumstances and experiences that shaped it, validate that it makes sense that the Inner Critic would take on this protective role.

Express appreciation for the Inner Critic's protective strategies and its positive intention to help you, even if they have manifested in harmful ways. In many cases, our Inner Critic took its form as a necessary survival strategy. We literally may not have survived without it. If this is the case, make sure to let the Inner Critic know you see and understand this background.

Keep acknowledging and validating this part as long as needed, without necessarily agreeing with its methods and ways of relating to you. The Inner Critic might easily receive your validation and appreciation, or it might be skeptical, since it's probably not used to having a conversation with your Self-energy. Let it know that any resistance, distrust or skepticism is OK and understandable. This part doesn't have to fully trust you right away. Stay steady in your validation until it starts to receive what you are saying, even if only a little.

E Educate

Now you are going to educate the Inner Critic to update it to the present, as well as to teach it what role it can play that is most supportive to you.

Educate the Inner Critic about your current reality. It is extremely common for an Inner Critic to believe you are younger than you actually are or for it not to know that you are no longer in the circumstances in which it originally arose. The Inner Critic may also know you are an adult, but it may mistake the fullness of who you are for certain parts of you, particularly parts it judges as unacceptable or unreliable.

Ask the Inner Critic how old it thinks you are. If it thinks you are younger than you are, let it know how old you are and that you are an adult now. Let it know that you are no longer in the same circumstances that necessitated its presence. Describe your current life context and even show it what your life is like now.

Educate it about the impact of its methods. Again, acknowledge the Inner Critic's positive intentions and its role in trying to protect you. Express appreciation for its efforts to keep you safe and motivated. Then highlight the gap between what it's trying to do and how its approach has affected you. Share that you're not trying to shame or guilt the Inner Critic for how it has shown up. Instead, you're naming the mismatch between its intentions and the actual impact of its actions. Let it know that its way of relating to you has been unhelpful, even harmful or paralyzing.

U Update

Now update the Inner Critic so that it inhabits the present and functions in a supportive role. This process involves updating its understanding of your present circumstances and guiding it toward more constructive ways to help you.

- **Establish a new inner authority.** Let the part know that *you*—your present-moment, adult Self—are now in charge. You are responsible for making decisions, setting boundaries and navigating life. Even if you're still learning or growing, Self is leading now.
- **Explore its wishes.** Ask the Inner Critic if it still wants to serve as a protector in some way, or if it feels ready to rest, retire, transform or even dissolve. Some parts may want a new role; others may long to be free of responsibility altogether. Listen with curiosity.
- **Clarify a new role (if desired).** If the Critic does want to stay, invite it to become an Inner Coach—an updated version of itself that still holds its positive intentions for you but offers clear guidance and encouragement instead of criticism. Suggest ways it might offer support without using fear or pressure. Frame this as an evolution—not a rejection—of its original purpose.
- **Propose new methods.** Offer some specific examples of how it could help you in healthier ways, like encouraging you with affirming reminders, prompting reflection before reacting, offering clear and constructive feedback, or helping you prioritize self-care and boundaries.
- **Ask what it needs.** Before any shift can happen, ask what this part needs to feel safe making the change. Does it need reassurance, practice, trust or a specific kind of

support from you or other parts? Let it know that you're willing to collaborate.
- **Close with appreciation.** Thank this part for its long service and dedication, even if its methods have been painful. Let it know you'll return to keep deepening this relationship.

What to Do Next

After this initial conversation, you must reinforce the changes by consistently reminding the Inner Critic of its new role. Our suggestion is to take on these practices as often as you need to in order to experience and reinforce the Inner Critic's transformation. This may be every few days, weeks or months, or on an as-needed basis. The following suggestions can also be applied to your other Shame Triangle parts.

Remind Your Inner Critic of the Changes

This practice will help solidify the changes and strengthen your Inner Coach's ability to guide you with more encouragement and wisdom. By consistently connecting with this part and reminding it of its updated role, you can gradually rewire its old patterns. Here is a practice you can use on a regular basis to help reinforce the new role of your Inner Coach:
- Set aside a few minutes each day to connect with your newly transformed Inner Coach (formerly the Inner Critic).
- First, center in Self and then visualize or imagine your Inner Coach standing before you. Greet this part warmly, acknowledging its presence in your life and expressing gratitude for how it has tried to protect you over the years, even if its methods were misguided or were right for the past, but are no longer helpful in the present.
- Remind your Inner Coach that its old harsh, critical ways are no longer helpful or necessary. You can again

point out that you are now an adult, no longer in the same circumstances that originally gave rise to this part's protective strategies.
- Reinforce the new role and job description you have cocreated for your Inner Coach. Remind it of how you need it to function now, as a supportive guide.
- If you know a situation is coming up that would typically activate the old version of your Inner Critic, you can let it know beforehand what would be most helpful. Tell it your expectations for communicating with you and how you would like it to show up as an Inner Coach.

Translate, Translate, Translate!

Our Inner Critic is used to doing things its own way, so change doesn't happen overnight. When its old, familiar voice shows up, pause. Then ask it to *translate*—to speak to you as an Inner Coach, rather than a harsh critic. Think of it like training a puppy. Just as we gently and consistently remind a puppy not to jump up or bite, we need to redirect the Inner Critic when it slips back into its old patterns. This isn't about punishment—it's about repetition, guidance and patience. Over time, the part can learn a new way of relating.

Sometimes, a simple prompt is enough for the part to shift. Other times, it might hesitate or resist. If asking it to translate doesn't work, don't force it. Instead, pause, reconnect with Self and reflect on what this part is really trying to offer you. Even if its delivery is harsh, its intention is often rooted in protection, care or motivation. You don't have to engage the criticism directly—instead, you can translate the message yourself by tuning in to the deeper need it points to. Then ask: How can I give myself that now—in a way that's truly supportive?

- **Throughout your day, stay attuned to the voice of your Inner Critic.** When you notice its old familiar tone, pause.

- **From Self, kindly interrupt**: "Ah, that's the old way. Please speak to me as an Inner Coach instead."

These first two steps are often enough to shift the energy. If not, keep going:
- **If the part can't find its new voice yet, that's OK.** Take a few breaths to reconnect with Self. Let the part know it doesn't have to force anything right now. Ask it to step back gently, so you can listen for what it really needs.
- **Reflect on the part's deeper positive intention.** Is it trying to help you succeed? Protect you from harm? Earn acceptance? Express care? Then ask: What would safety, growth or love look like in this moment? How can I give that to myself right now?
- **Bring that energy into the present.** Offer yourself the encouragement, clarity or compassion this part is truly trying to provide. Let that energy guide your response to the situation at hand.
- **Thank the part for showing up.** Let it know that this is an ongoing process, and you'll be back to keep building trust. You're not trying to get rid of the part—you're working with it. Change takes time, and you're in it together.

Be patient and persistent. This translation process may need to happen a hundred times before it becomes second nature. Celebrate small wins! Every time you catch the critical voice and redirect it, you are rewiring it.

Transforming Shame

Now that you have worked with your Inner Critic, your Shame should have some necessary breathing room. Facing Shame can be challenging, and it's understandable if you feel hesitant. You might fear that by moving toward it, you'll confirm the harsh judgments of the Inner Critic or uncover something unbearable about yourself. You may worry that the pain Shame holds will overwhelm you. If you have these fears, you are not alone. But by approaching Shame from Self, you won't find proof of unworthiness—you'll find a part of yourself in need of love, care and connection.

Among the three parts of the Shame Triangle, Shame carries our deepest pain. It often holds negative beliefs about our worth, value and lovability, shaped by the ways we were once dismissed, mistreated or silenced. Because of this background, it is essential to stay unblended and centered in the caring, connected qualities of Self. Similar to the Inner Critic, Shame can be deeply convincing. It will point to past experiences—things we've done, things done to us or injustices in the world—as proof that we are deficient or undeserving of compassion. But this perspective is a function of the Shame Triangle, not Self. Even if we have made mistakes or caused harm, we are still worthy of being free from the cycle of self-condemnation.

Before you begin a dialogue with your Shame, it's important to recognize that it isn't just one thing. Shame holds a wound, but it also protects us. Most discussions of parts holding shame focus on it as an exiled inner child, but Shame is also a protector. It tries to keep us safe by making us small, compliant or invisible, encouraging us to appease, submit or avoid confrontation to prevent further harm. It keeps us from expressing ourselves fully, standing up for our needs or embracing our uniqueness— believing that staying under the radar is the safest path.

At its core, Shame is trying to maintain our belonging. Just as fear protects us from physical danger, Shame alerts us when our social standing feels at risk. It warns us of the possibility of judgment, exclusion or failure, making it one of the most deeply relational parts of our system. The pain of rejection is real, but so are the added burdens Shame creates in its attempt to prevent possible rejection. Because Shame acts as both a wounded part and a protector—a wounded warrior—we must meet it on both levels: acknowledging its pain while also understanding how it has tried to shield us.

Self LOVE U Shame Process

In this section, we will again use the Self LOVE U process we used with the Inner Critic, but we will adapt it slightly to meet the needs of our Shame part. As you'll see, in the process for Shame, the E in Self LOVE U focuses more on *embracing* than *educating*. In this first encounter, aim to get to know Shame and its history, and relate to it in ways that show it you are an ally and can be trusted. You are establishing a relationship between this part and Self. After you've connected with Shame, remember there is more unburdening to come in later chapters.

- **Self** Connect with Self-Energy
- **L** Locate Shame
- **O** Origin Story
- **V** Validate Its Experiences
- **E** Embrace
- **U** Update

Self Connect with Self-Energy

Close your eyes and turn inward. Take a few deep breaths, letting each exhale settle you into the present moment. Allow yourself to sink into Self-energy. If any parts are active, kindly ask them to step back for now. However, sometimes the Inner Critic would like to be present for this process. If so, let your Inner Critic know that it can watch, but not jump in. The goal here is to stay curious, engaged and open while dialoguing with your Shame.

L Locate Shame

The key to this step is to connect to Self-energy and then create an internal separation between Self and Shame, allowing you to have a dialogue and better understand this part of you without blending with it.

Once centered and grounded, locate your Shame within your physical or psychological space. Where does it show up? Pay attention to whether it manifests as a feeling inside your body, a voice inside your head or an external presence around you.

If you experience Shame inside your body or mind, invite it to externalize by stepping outside of you. Imagine it taking a form and positioning itself at a comfortable distance in front of you. The externalized Shame may appear as a clear humanlike figure, a younger version of yourself or an abstract form. You also might experience it through intuition, sound or a felt sense rather than visually.

Let this part know you are here to connect with it. If Shame is hesitant to engage or resistant to externalizing, reassure it that you are not trying to get rid of it or punish it. Explain that your intention is simply to connect with and understand it better, and it can return to you after the conversation.

Once Shame is externalized, take a moment to feel the space between you and this part. Maintain an open, curious stance toward Shame. If any other parts jump in, kindly ask them to step aside and assure them that you are in Self, which can handle talking to Shame.

O   Origin Story

Begin getting to know your Shame by asking about its origin story. How long has this part been with you? What life circumstances created it? When did it first appear? What events or experiences contributed to its development? What does it feel is important for you to know now? Remember to listen from Self without reliving the part's experiences. If Shame overwhelms you, ask it to slow down or imagine it smaller or farther away. You can also project it onto a screen or phone to watch from a safe distance.

Next, inquire about the wounds Shame holds. What is the core wound that Shame holds about itself? What are the beliefs it took on because of this wound? Are there any recurring themes or patterns in the beliefs that Shame holds because of this wound? How does Shame cope with the pain of this wound on a day-to-day basis? Does Shame desire healing or resolution for this wound (even if it doesn't know how to achieve it)?

Once you get a good sense of how and why this part came about, inquire about Shame's intentions, purpose, role or job. Ask: What does this part want for you? What job or role has it taken on? What is it trying to protect you from? What is its intention for you? What is it trying to achieve? How does it believe it's helping you? If Shame states its intention negatively by saying what it doesn't want for you or what it's trying to avoid (e.g., to keep you from getting hurt or to avoid abandonment), continue to inquire into those motivations until you get to its positive intention (e.g., it wants you to be loved, accepted or safe). Understanding this protective intention is pivotal to transforming your relationship with Shame.

V   Validate Its Experiences

In this step, validate your Shame part by acknowledging the challenges and difficulties it has endured on your behalf. Let it know you get it, you understand. With as much sincerity as you can muster, acknowledge how hard it's been for this part up until now. Let this part know that you see it and that you've heard it. Let this part know you truly recognize the hardship, pain, confusion and trauma it has been through. Recognize that, based on what this part has gone through, its feelings and beliefs make perfect sense. Validate that what it went through was not its fault and that it's not responsible for how it was treated by others.

Express appreciation for Shame's protective role and its positive intention to help you, even if that help has manifested in harmful ways. In many cases, Shame takes its form as a survival strategy, and we literally may not have survived without it. If this is the case, make sure to let Shame know you see and understand this background now. Keep acknowledging and validating this part as long as needed, without necessarily agreeing with its methods or beliefs. Shame might easily receive your validation and appreciation, or it might be skeptical, since it's probably not used to having a conversation with your Self-energy. Let it know that any resistance, distrust or skepticism is OK and understandable. Stay steady in your validation until it starts to receive what you are saying, even if only a little.

E Embrace

Typically, after you validate and acknowledge Shame's experience and intent, you will see a shift in its posture or energy. It may relax, expand, express gratitude or even take a different form. The Embrace step is about going a level deeper with your validation of the part by connecting from your heart. Ask Shame about its feelings and what it has been holding onto. Ask it about its needs and longings. Listen closely and pay special attention to needs for love, connection, authenticity and autonomy, as well as needs to matter, to be seen, to be understood or to be protected. If your part states that its need is for the absence of something, for someone else to do something specific or for someone to be different in some way, you can inquire further by asking, "What need would that change fulfill?" Once you are able to identify its core needs, embrace this part and offer it what it needs.

When embracing Shame, you can imagine literally holding it, hugging it or offering to hold its hand. You can imagine love or light extending from your heart outward toward it. You can imagine that this part is being embraced by a loved one (alive or passed), an archetypal figure or an angelic being. You can imagine that you are being embraced by an aspect of nature such as a tree, rays of sunlight, ocean waves or the earth itself. If nothing occurs to you at the moment, you can also ask the part directly how it would like you to embrace and support it. You may be surprised by what it tells you. This part of the process is known as inner reparenting, and there's no "right" way to do it. Simply do whatever works best for you and for this part. Trust the wisdom of your inner system when it tells you what it needs to feel embraced. By extending empathy and embracing your Shame part, you are giving it the love, care and understanding it previously lacked. This embrace helps to heal Shame's wounds and transforms this part from a source of pain into a part that embodies tender vulnerability and care.

U   Update

Now update Shame so that it inhabits the present. Ask the part how old it thinks you are and if it knows you are an adult. Make it aware of your current circumstances and that you are now an adult, no longer in the original conditions that brought it into being. If Shame is still in the past, imagine bringing it into the present moment with you. You can visualize a time-lapse or movie montage of your life, showing it the growth and changes you have experienced. Walk it around your home or life, pointing out key aspects of your current reality. If needed, imagine airlifting it out of the past into the present, giving it a clear view of your present-day circumstances. And if the part doesn't want to live in your current reality, that's OK—it may prefer to settle into an entirely different inner place, somewhere it feels free, light and unburdened.

Once the part has been updated—whether to your current reality or a place where it feels free—it's important to establish a new relationship with it. Let the part know that you can handle its feelings now—that whatever arises, you're here to be with it, not to push it away. Let it know that you, as Self, are leading and responsible for creating healthy boundaries among your parts and in your life. Reassure it that your present-moment adult self is capable of making decisions, navigating relationships and staying grounded through difficult emotions. Clarify that it no longer has to protect you by shrinking, hiding or blaming yourself. Instead of filtering your experience through the lens of unworthiness, this part can begin to simply *be*—allowing your Raw Experience to move through without judgment or story. If this part starts to slip back into old shame storylines, gently guide it back to the truth: You are safe to feel what you feel, and belonging is not something you have to earn.

Ask Shame if there's anything else it wants you to know or if there's anything it needs from you before you close. Listen with patience, letting it express whatever arises. Once the conversation feels complete, thank it for sharing with you and for its willingness to be seen. Let it know that you'll be back to connect again, and that it doesn't have to hold everything alone. When you're ready, take a deep breath, gently bring your awareness back to the present moment and close the exercise.

Transforming Escapers

Our Escapers aim to protect us from danger, both real and perceived. Like professional escape artists who navigate fire, locked chains and submerged boxes, our Escapers react to the metaphorical handcuffs, straitjackets and nailed coffins of our lives. They work creatively to keep us from feeling trapped, finding ways to avoid the emotional and psychological pain that threatens our sense of self.

Our Escapers also work to protect us from the uncomfortable. While we are born with the capacity to experience a full range of emotions, our upbringing and culture condition us to tolerate only a narrow spectrum. When we encounter emotions deemed negative or unacceptable, we dissociate from them. However, the energy of our Raw Experiences doesn't simply vanish. Instead, the Escapers transmute it into busyness, numbing, aggression or self-harm. While these avoidance strategies may initially seem protective or temporarily effective, they can lead to long-term emotional and psychological consequences, as unresolved emotions continue to influence our behavior beneath the surface.

One of my favorite allegories about Escapers comes from Anita Johnston's book *Eating in the Light of the Moon* (2000), in which she tells a story about a girl who falls into a raging river. Struggling to stay afloat, the girl grabs onto a log. The log saves her from drowning. But when she is finally downstream in calmer waters and tries to reach the riverbank, she finds she can't pull herself up out of the water. Clinging to the log, she is unable to reach solid ground. The very thing that saved her is now keeping her stuck. The log is too big and heavy to lift onto the shore, so she would have to let it go in order to climb out of the river and reach the safety of land.

This is how Escapers function: They protect us when we need them, but can later hold us back. Just as the girl must eventually release the log to step onto the riverbank, we must release outdated survival strategies when they no longer serve us. Transforming our Escapers into Inner Nurturers—parts that turn toward discomfort rather than away—allows us to meet our emotions with care, rather than avoidance. Instead of numbing, distracting or overcompensating, we can learn to sit with our experience, process what arises and offer ourselves the comfort and regulation we actually need. This shift helps us engage with life from a place of resilience rather than reactivity, making space for genuine healing and growth.

Self LOVE U Escaper Process

Just as you did with the Inner Critic and Shame, you will now connect with your Escaper through the Self LOVE U process.

Self	Connect with Self-Energy
L	Locate the Escaper
O	Origin Story
V	Validate Its Efforts and Intentions
E	Educate
U	Update

Self   Connect with Self-Energy

Close your eyes and turn inward. Take a few deep breaths, letting each exhale settle you into the present moment. If any parts are active, kindly ask them to step back for now. Allow yourself to relax into Self-energy. Rest here for a few moments, or longer if needed, until you feel centered and ready to begin. Take your time to ensure a solid grounding in your Self-energy before moving on to the "Locate" step.

L   Locate the Escaper

Once centered and grounded, locate your Escaper within your physical or psychological space. Where does it show up? Pay attention to whether it manifests as a voice inside your head, a feeling within your body or an external presence around you.

If you experience the Escaper inside your body or mind, invite it to externalize by stepping outside of you. Imagine it taking a form and positioning itself at a comfortable distance in front of you. The externalized Escaper may appear as a clear humanlike figure, a younger version of yourself or an abstract form. You might also experience this part through intuition, sound or a felt sense rather than visually.

If the Escaper is hesitant to engage or resistant to externalizing, reassure it that you are not trying to get rid of it or punish it. Explain that your intention is simply to connect with and understand it better. Once it's externalized, observe the Escaper's characteristics—its voice, body language, facial expressions, color, texture, overall feel, etc. Notice any feelings or sensations that arise as you engage with this externalized part of yourself.

Maintain an open, curious stance toward the Escaper. If any other parts jump in, kindly ask them to step aside and reassure them that you are in Self, which can handle talking to the Escaper.

O   Origin Story

Begin getting to know your Escaper by asking about its origin story. How long has this part been with you? What life circumstances created this part? When did it first appear? What events or experiences contributed to its development? Ask the part what it feels is important for you to know now.

Once you get a good sense of how and why this part came about, inquire about the Escaper's intentions, purpose, role or job. Ask: What does this part want for you? What job or role has it taken on? What is it trying to protect you from? What is its intention for you? What is it trying to achieve? How does it believe it's helping you?

If the Escaper states its intention negatively, continue to inquire until you get to its positive intention.

V Validate Its Efforts and Intentions

After getting the Escaper's story and understanding the role it's played, validate and acknowledge this part for how it came about and why it took its particular form. Acknowledge that the Escaper has been trying to keep you safe. Express appreciation for the Escaper's protective role and its positive intention to help you, even if it has manifested in harmful ways.

Validate the Escaper's experiences and the challenges it has endured on your behalf. Validate how it makes sense, given the circumstances and experiences that shaped it, that the Escaper would take on this protective role. Keep acknowledging and validating this part as long as needed, without necessarily agreeing with its methods and ways of relating to you. The Escaper might easily receive your validation and appreciation, or it might be skeptical, since it's probably not used to having a conversation with your Self-energy. Let it know that any resistance, distrust or skepticism is OK and understandable. Stay steady in your validation until it starts to receive what you are saying, even if only a little.

E Educate

After you acknowledge the Escaper's positive intentions and its role in trying to protect you, and express appreciation for its efforts to keep you safe, it's time to highlight the discrepancy between its intentions and its ways of relating to you. Explain that you're not trying to shame or guilt the Escaper for how it has shown up. Instead, you're inviting it to consider how its strategies—though well-meaning—have often caused harm or led to outcomes neither of you truly want. Let it know that its patterns of avoiding, numbing or appeasing haven't helped you move toward the deeper safety, connection or freedom it's actually been trying to create.

U   Update

Ask the Escaper how old it thinks you are and if it knows you are an adult. Make it aware of your current circumstances and that you are now an adult, no longer in the original conditions that brought it into being. If the Escaper is stuck in the past, imagine bringing it into the present moment with you. Visualize a time-lapse or movie montage of your life, showing the growth and changes you have experienced. Walk it around your home or life, pointing out key aspects of your current reality. If needed, imagine airlifting it out of the past into the present, giving it a clear view of your present-day circumstances.

Let the Escaper know that you—your present-moment adult Self—are now in charge. You're responsible for setting boundaries, making decisions and handling what life brings. Reassure it that it no longer has to carry that weight alone. Once this new relationship is established, invite the Escaper to consider a new role—one that still honors its original purpose but uses different methods. Instead of avoiding discomfort, what if it could help you face difficult feelings with care? What if it could support you by helping you slow down, check in and stay connected to what matters? If it's ready, guide the Escaper in transforming into an Inner Nurturer—a part that helps you regulate, rest and respond to emotion rather than run from it. You might offer gentle ideas for how it could help now: reminding you to take a break before overwhelm hits, prompting self-compassion when you're hurting or encouraging emotional connection rather than escape. Let it know this is a process, and it doesn't have to be perfect. You'll keep listening and adjusting together as you go.

Thank this part. Ask if it needs anything else to feel complete for now. When you're ready, take a moment to shift out of the conversation, bring your attention back to your surroundings and return to the present moment.

∆

The conversation between Self and your parts has begun. And like in every good relationship, it will continue. It will deepen, shift and surprise you. Some parts will step easily into new roles, relieved to be heard and freed from jobs they no longer need to do. Others might hesitate, uncertain of what comes next, needing patience and reassurance before they let go. That's OK. There is no rush. What matters is that you keep showing up—listening, responding and leading with Self. Now, we turn to the next chapters, where we will fortify our shift from the Shame Triangle to the Self-Love Triangle by applying the Self-centered model to our body, heart and mind.

CHAPTER 7
THE SHAME TRIANGLE AND THE BODY

In this chapter, we turn our attention to how the Shame Triangle lives in the body and affects our ability to stay grounded and regulated. It isn't just a pattern of thoughts or emotions. It shows up in our posture, breath, tension and movement. The nervous system may register the voices of our Inner Critic, Shame or Escapers as threats, triggering protective reactions or survival responses in the body. At the same time, these parts can be expressions of dysregulation—emerging when the system is overwhelmed and trying to regain a sense of control or safety. Because the body, heart and mind are deeply interconnected, what happens in the body affects everything. Dysregulation in the body can ripple outward, spreading to the other centers—creating waves of emotional overwhelm in the heart and stirring up harsh narratives in the mind—and drowning out Self-energy in the process.

The Shame Triangle intersects with the body in many ways. We could explore body image, eating disorders, chronic pain, illness or exhaustion. Each of these impacts deserves careful attention. But underneath them all lies a core issue: the body's ability to regulate itself. Without that capacity, it's difficult to engage the Shame Triangle in a meaningful way—regardless of what story or struggle it's tied to. That's why this chapter focuses on dysregulation: what it is, how the Shame Triangle activates it, and what it takes to restore a felt sense of safety, connection and balance in the body.

The Shame Triangle and Nervous System Survival Responses

When the Shame Triangle is active, the body shifts into a survival state. The nervous system perceives a threat—whether physical, emotional or social—and responds automatically. This isn't theoretical; it's biological. Early experiences of shame, exclusion or ridicule become imprinted in the body's stress response. Over time, the body learns that certain feelings, expressions or even ways of being are unsafe. In response, it activates defenses like withdrawal, numbing, appeasement or internal attack—locking us into patterns of survival that are hard to break.

To understand how this reaction shows up in the body, we turn to the Four F's of survival: fight, flight, freeze and fawn. Originally introduced as the fight-or-flight model by physiologist Walter Bradford Cannon in the early 20th century, this framework was expanded in the 1960s and '70s by trauma researchers such as Bessel van der Kolk and Stephen Porges to include the freeze response, which involves shutdown and dissociation. In 2013, Pete Walker added the fawn response to describe how people-pleasing and appeasement can also function as survival strategies. Each of these responses has a distinct physiological pattern:
- **Fight:** The body prepares to confront a threat. Heart rate spikes, muscles tighten and adrenaline surges—readying us for action, whether physical or verbal.
- **Flight:** The body mobilizes to escape. Energy surges toward movement, thoughts race and we feel a strong

urge to flee—either by physically leaving or mentally checking out.
- **Freeze:** The body shuts down. Breathing slows, muscles go limp and everything feels distant or heavy. In certain cases, the freeze state leads to dissociation.
- **Fawn:** The body moves to appease. Muscles may tense in anticipation of others' reactions, breath may become shallow, and the nervous system shifts into a heightened state of social vigilance. To avoid conflict, rejection or shame, we suppress our own needs and emotions in order to maintain safety or connection—often by over-accommodating others.

Each part of the Shame Triangle may express one or more of the survival responses. These patterns can shift from person to person, and even from moment to moment, depending on context and what the nervous system perceives as threatening. While we'll explore how each part often maps onto specific defenses, these are not fixed categories. Despite the general patterns, only you can answer which survival response is most typical for each of your parts. Recognizing the nervous system's role in these patterns helps us respond more effectively. It allows us to see how these parts are not acting randomly or irrationally—they are responding to the body's perception of threat. When we understand how the body is trying to protect us, we can begin to work with it, creating conditions for safety, regulation and more Self-leadership.

The Inner Critic and the Fight Response Turned Inward

To the Inner Critic, anything that signals weakness—feeling inadequate, making mistakes, expressing emotions that seem like "too much" or falling short of expectations—is perceived as a direct threat to our survival. In response, it attacks those vulnerabilities, believing that criticism will protect us. The Inner Critic goes on the offensive, launching preemptive strikes against us, aiming to criticize us first before anyone else can. It tells us to push harder, so we'll never fall behind. Be perfect, and maybe we'll be safe. But this fight isn't against an external enemy—it's an internal war, one that keeps us in a constant state of tension, anxiety and self-doubt. What was meant to protect us only drains us, leaving us locked in battle with ourselves.

When this self-attack starts, the sympathetic nervous system responds as if we're facing an external threat. Our heart rate spikes, our muscles tighten, our breathing becomes shallow and our body braces for impact—even though the "enemy" is inside us (Halamová et al. 2019). This reaction mirrors the classic fight response, except instead of lashing out at others, we turn that aggression inward.

The Inner Critic often attacks with a force that is completely out of proportion to reality. This magnitude can create what we might call an autoimmune Shame Triangle flare-up: Much like an autoimmune disorder mistakenly attacks healthy cells, our Inner Critic turns our own physiological defenses against us. The very self-policing strategies meant to protect us end up tearing us down instead. Rather than keeping us safe, they drain our emotional and physical resources.

Living in a constant state of self-criticism takes a massive toll. The body was never meant to exist under perpetual attack. Over time, a chronic fight response can lead to burnout from mental pressure, chronic fatigue from staying stuck in high alert and increased inflammation due to prolonged stress hormone activation (Cwinn 2018). Studies have found that persistent self-attack increases cortisol levels, weakens immune function, and is linked to anxiety, depression and exhaustion (Lee 2005). Instead of safeguarding our well-being, the Inner Critic leaves us depleted, less able to handle challenges and more disconnected from ourselves and others.

This fight response also influences how we engage with the world. A chronically self-critical nervous system is stuck in a defensive posture, making it difficult to trust others, regulate emotions or be open to feedback (Rocha and Penido 2024). When our Inner Critic is on high alert, we anticipate problems before they happen, interpret neutral interactions as attacks and struggle to feel safe in relationships. We may seem overly sensitive to feedback, react defensively or shut down emotionally. Over time, these patterns erode connection and deepen isolation. Instead of protecting us, the Inner Critic limits our ability to fully engage with life. It traps us in cycles of tension, hypervigilance and self-doubt, keeping us from experiencing the very things it claims to protect—belonging, success and safety.

Reflection Questions

- When your Inner Critic is active, how does your body respond? Notice physical signs: Does your breath become shallow? Do you feel tension in your jaw, shoulders or stomach? How does your posture change?
- What are the long-term effects of living in a state of self-attack? Consider how chronic self-criticism might contribute to chronic conditions, exhaustion, stress or a sense of disconnection from yourself and your environment.
- How does being in a state of internal attack affect how you relate to others? When your body is tense and on guard, do you find yourself more reactive, defensive or withdrawn in relationships?

Shame and the Freeze Response

While the Inner Critic fuels the fight response by criticizing us, Shame pulls us in the opposite direction. It doesn't fight back. It doesn't try to run. Instead, it shuts us down completely. It doesn't activate the body with urgency and tension; it drains it. It strips away energy, numbs sensation and leaves us lethargic and collapsed. It's that sinking, suffocating feeling in the body that makes us want to disappear—shoulders hunched, head down, breath shallow. When Shame takes over, we freeze. We isolate. We withdraw from life, convinced we don't belong and that no one wants us anyway.

Freeze is a primal nervous system response. If the fight response is about proving ourselves and the flight response is about escaping judgment, the freeze response is about disappearing altogether. This is a physiological shutdown. When we're overwhelmed by shame, the nervous system shifts into freeze mode, slowing movement, numbing sensation and disconnecting us from both ourselves and the world around us (Porges 2003). The brain follows suit. The prefrontal cortex—the part responsible for rational thought, problem-solving and perspective-taking—goes offline. Meanwhile, the amygdala (our fear center) and brain stem survival circuits take control (Roelofs 2017).

This neurological shift blocks our ability to communicate and connect. We might struggle to form words. Our voice may flatten. Our mind goes blank. Eye contact might feel impossible. Research on the freeze response suggests that when the nervous system enters this state, our social engagement system is inhibited—we physically can't respond the way we normally would (Porges 2003). This is why, in moments of deep shame, even simple conversations feel unbearable. Someone might ask a genuine question, but we freeze—not because we don't want to respond, but because our body won't let us. It's also why we struggle to speak up for ourselves, set boundaries or express what we need.

In addition, the freeze response distorts our perception. Because higher brain functions are offline, we see the world through a narrow, fear-based lens. We misinterpret interactions, assume the worst and feel even more isolated (Roelofs et al. 2010). This is why shame-based shutdowns make it so hard to repair relationships—we literally lose access to the mental faculties that would help us see the bigger picture. Over time, repeated shame-induced freeze responses can condition us to believe that we are powerless to change—a phenomenon known as learned helplessness. This makes Shame one of the most paralyzing survival strategies.

> **Reflection Questions**

- Think of a recent situation where you felt overwhelmed by feelings of shame. What physical sensations did you notice in your body (e.g., changes in breathing, muscle tension, temperature)?
- When Shame arises, how does it affect your ability to move or speak? Do you notice any changes in your posture, voice or capacity to make eye contact?
- When Shame surfaces, do you shut down, withdraw or check out from the people around you? Do you disengage from conversations, activities or relationships?

Escapers and the Four F's

While the Inner Critic fights Shame head-on and Shame collapses under its weight, the Escaper has one goal: get away. It dodges, distracts and detours around discomfort. Depending on the situation, it speeds up, slows down, lashes out or disappears entirely. It fuels busyness, aggression, withdrawal or compliance, all in service of one goal: staying ahead of Shame.

When the nervous system is in hyperarousal, the Escaper shifts into overdrive, trying to control or outrun emotional pain. Some parts escape through flight—filling every moment with activity, chasing productivity or perfecting every detail. The body stays tense, the mind races and exhaustion feels like the price of being enough. If there's no room for stillness, there's no space for Shame to creep in. Other parts try to fight their way out. Instead of feeling small, they puff up, lash out, criticize or blame. The goal isn't cruelty; it's protection. The more they attack, the less they have to feel the sting of self-doubt. But anger turned outward can just as easily turn inward. When there's no one else to fight, the target becomes the self—through self-harm, reckless behavior, numbing substances or risky choices, each one an attempt to override Shame, punish failure or momentarily feel in control (Brown 2012; Kaufman 1989).

But when fight and flight seem impossible, the Escaper shuts down. It numbs out, disconnects or disintegrates into the void. Motivation drains away, responsibilities pile up and even small tasks feel insurmountable. The body slows, the world feels distant and time blurs at the edges. A pull toward mindless distractions takes over—endless scrolling, binge-watching, anything to dull the weight of existing. For some, this withdrawal feels like relief, but underneath, it deepens helplessness, making it even harder to re-engage (Maté 2010; van der Kolk 2014).

One of the most deceptive forms of escaping, though, isn't running, fighting or shutting down—it's appeasing. Some parts of us learn that the safest way to survive the Inner Critic and Shame is to stay small, agreeable and pleasing. If they keep others happy, they might be OK. If they apologize first, maybe they won't be blamed. If they anticipate every need, maybe they'll be indispensable. These parts don't just try to escape shame; they try to earn worthiness. But the cost is steep: the further they bend, the more they lose themselves (Gilligan 1982; Neff 2003).

These responses aren't rigid—they shift based on safety, power dynamics and conditioning. If one escape strategy fails—perhaps exciting the Inner Critic or Shame too quickly—we instinctively switch to another. If numbing out with social media doesn't dull discomfort enough, we might throw ourselves into overworking instead. If humor won't diffuse tension in a workplace setting, we might default to people-pleasing. The strategy we use depends on the context and what feels most accessible in the moment. This constant shifting isn't random—it reflects the body's ongoing attempt to secure safety in real time (Levine 1997; Schauer et al. 2011; Walker 2013).

Cultural and social conditioning also shape which escape patterns become dominant. While everyone has access to all four survival strategies, societal expectations reinforce certain responses over others. Women, for instance, are often socialized to appease—prioritizing harmony over confrontation (Gilligan 1982). Men, on the other hand, are more likely to externalize distress through anger or withdrawal, and are discouraged from expressing vulnerability (Breslau et al. 1991). Similarly, people raised in authoritarian households may have learned that fighting back is dangerous, but appeasement ensures safety, while those from unpredictable environments may have developed the ability to rapidly switch between strategies depending on the situation. These learned patterns persist into adulthood, even when the original threats are gone (Maté 2003; Porges 2011), shaping how our Shame Triangle Escapers react.

Reflection Questions

- How does your body feel when your Escaper takes over? Do you notice tension, restlessness, numbness or a shift in energy? Where in your body do you feel it most—your chest, stomach, shoulders or elsewhere?
- What nervous system state do you most often default to? Do you fawn? Do you tend to speed up into hyperarousal (fight or flight) or shut down into hypoarousal (freeze)? Or do you shift between them?
- What physical cues signal that you're in an Escaper state? Do you find yourself clenching your jaw, holding your breath, feeling jittery, collapsing into exhaustion or zoning out? How does your posture, breathing or movement change?
- When your Escaper activates, do you reach for movement, stillness, stimulation or avoidance? Which of these patterns seem to bring relief, and which leave you feeling more dysregulated?

Regulating the Four F Responses of the Nervous System

All of these patterns start as protection, but over time, they become prisons. Running never leads to rest. Lashing out never brings relief. Numbing out never creates peace. Appeasing never guarantees love. Our Escapers ultimately want to keep us safe, but real safety comes not from escaping ourselves, but from turning toward what we've been running from (Neff 2021).

Turning toward isn't just a mental or emotional shift—it's a physiological one. Each defense response affects the nervous system differently and requires different strategies to bring the body back into regulation. The following exercises are designed to engage the body directly to shift it out of dysregulation. Some will help you release excess energy, some bring grounding and containment, and others gently awaken the system from shutdown. Your task isn't to force a change, but to experiment and notice what resonates, what soothes and what helps you reclaim a sense of Self-led inner steadiness.

Regulating the Fight Response

When the fight response is activated, the body is on high alert, tense and prepared for battle. This often leads to anger, frustration, irritation or rage. If this energy has nowhere to go, it can turn inward as harsh self-judgment or outward as irritability toward others. The goal of these exercises is to discharge pent-up energy safely while restoring a sense of ease and control. While several of these exercises are described from standing, if you are unable to stand or move your legs, you can do them with your upper body.

The Grounding Push

The tension of the fight response can create an energy buildup in the body. This exercise provides a controlled and safe way to push that energy out of your system.
- Stand with your feet firmly planted, hip-width apart.
- Place your hands on a sturdy surface (wall, countertop or desk).
- Push against it with all your strength for five to ten seconds, engaging your muscles.
- As you push, imagine releasing tension and criticism outward.
- Make any noise you'd like to assist with this release.
- Exhale deeply and slowly release the push.
- Repeat two or three times, then shake out your arms and legs to discharge the remaining energy.

Ecstatic Shaking

The fight response locks the body in a state of tightness and rigidity. Shaking is a biological reset mechanism found in nature—animals instinctively shake after a stressful event to discharge adrenaline and return to a calm state. This practice helps the nervous system release stored stress and tension (Levine 2010).
- Stand in a comfortable space with your feet grounded.
- Begin bouncing gently on your feet, shaking out your arms and legs.
- Gradually increase the intensity—let your whole body shake, even your head and shoulders.
- If it feels natural, let out a sigh, hum or vocalization to enhance the release.
- Shake for three to five minutes, then gradually slow down.
- Stand still, take deep breaths and notice how your body feels.

Pillow Punching

This exercise offers a safe, physical outlet for pent-up fight energy or a way to release anger or frustration in the moment.
- Find a pillow or punching bag.
- Take deep breaths, feeling your feet grounded.
- Using slow, controlled movements, punch the pillow while exhaling forcefully.
- If helpful, vocalize sounds (a grunt or "HA!") to further release tension.
- Continue for a minute or two, then pause and notice how your body feels.

The Primal Roar

The fight response can build up intense energy in the body, creating an urge to yell or release sound. This exercise provides a controlled way to discharge tension through vocalization, engaging the diaphragm and vagus nerve (which is responsible for calming the nervous system and regulating stress responses) to help reset the nervous system. By releasing a forceful roar or yell, you discharge stress, clear pent-up frustration, signal safety to your brain and regain a sense of power and control, ultimately restoring calm after a fight response activation.
- Find a private space where you feel comfortable making noise—indoors or outdoors.
- Stand with feet hip-width apart, knees slightly bent.
- Inhale deeply through your nose, expanding your belly.
- Exhale with a powerful roar, yell or "HA!" to release tension.
- Engage your whole body—stomp, punch the air or tighten fists as needed.
- Repeat three to five times, then breathe deeply and notice the shift in energy.

Regulating the Flight Response

When the flight response is activated, the nervous system is flooded with excess energy, racing thoughts and restlessness. You may feel jittery and unable to sit still. You might feel a strong urge to escape, whether physically by leaving or mentally by dissociating into thoughts or distractions. This response often leaves people feeling untethered, anxious or overstimulated. The aim of flight regulation exercises is to foster a sense of containment, grounding and stability to help slow the nervous system down.

5-4-3-2-1 Grounding

When the nervous system is stuck in flight, it moves too fast for the present moment. The 5-4-3-2-1 exercise helps anchor your awareness of what is real, reducing feelings of overwhelm (Rothschild 2000).
- Take a deep breath and exhale slowly.
- Identify:
  - **Five** things you can see.
  - **Four** things you can touch.
  - **Three** things you can hear.
  - **Two** things you can smell.
  - **One** thing you can taste.
- Breathe deeply again and notice how your body starts to settle.

Box Breathing (4-4-4-4)

Controlled breathing directly regulates the nervous system. The flight response speeds up breathing, keeping the body in a hyperactive state. Box breathing slows the heart rate, regulates oxygen flow and supports relaxation (Porges 2011). This exercise can also be used for the fight response before or after discharging fight energy.

- Inhale deeply through the nose for four seconds.
- Hold your breath for four seconds.
- Exhale slowly through the mouth for four seconds.
- Hold again for four seconds.
- Repeat for a few cycles, feeling your body calm.

Weighted Pressure Hold

When the nervous system is in flight mode, the body feels too activated to settle. You may feel jittery, restless or like you need to do something constantly. Deep pressure techniques help signal safety to the body by providing physical containment, which counteracts the sense of being untethered or "too fast." Research on deep pressure therapy (van der Kolk 2014) has shown that firm, consistent pressure on the body helps reduce anxiety and promote a calming parasympathetic nervous system response. This exercise can also help with the fight and fawn responses.

- If available, drape a weighted blanket over your shoulders or wrap yourself tightly in a regular blanket or large towel.
- If you don't have a blanket or towel, give yourself a compression hold:
  - Cross your arms over your chest and gently squeeze your shoulders.
  - Hold the position for a few seconds, breathing deeply.
  - Slowly move down, squeezing your upper arms, then forearms, then hands.
- Allow your body to register the sense of being held and supported.
- Continue as long as it feels soothing, then release and notice how your body feels.

Eye-Tracking Exercise (Orienting Response Reset)

The orienting response is a biological survival mechanism that allows the nervous system to assess whether an environment is safe or dangerous. When something moves in our peripheral vision, our eyes automatically track it. This response is embedded in the brain stem and is designed to keep us alert to potential threats. In hyperaroused states (like the flight response), the orienting response can become overactive, leading to constant scanning, difficulty focusing and a sense of being "on edge." This is because the brain remains stuck in a loop of hypervigilance, searching for danger even when none is present.

By intentionally engaging the eye muscles in slow, controlled tracking, you can reset the orienting response, interrupt the hypervigilant scanning and activate the parasympathetic nervous system (Schauer et al. 2011). This practice helps bring a sense of focus, stability and calm. It tells the brain that the environment has been fully scanned and found safe, allowing the nervous system to return to a regulated state.

- Sit in a comfortable position where you can keep your head still.
- Hold your finger, a pen or a small object at eye level, about a foot away from your face.
- Slowly move the object from left to right, following it only with your eyes (keep your head still).
- Move the object as far to the left as possible, then slowly bring it back across your field of vision to the far right.
- Repeat this movement five to ten times, breathing slowly.
- Close your eyes for a few seconds and notice if you feel more settled or grounded.

Regulating the Freeze Response

When the freeze response is activated, the body may feel numb, heavy or disconnected. Breathing slows, muscles may go limp, and the world can feel far away or unreal. This state often leads to feelings of helplessness, shame or dissociation. The goal of these exercises is to gently reawaken sensation, invite movement, and support a safe reconnection with your body and surroundings without overwhelming the system.

Humming or Vagal Toning

The vagus nerve controls the body's relaxation response. When freeze mode is active, vagal stimulation can help gently shift the nervous system out of shutdown (Porges 2011).
- Take a deep breath.
- Hum or make a low "mmmm" sound as you exhale.
- Feel the vibration in your throat and chest.
- Repeat several times, noticing any shifts in your awareness.

Gentle Rocking or Rhythmic Movement

Gentle, rhythmic motion mimics early soothing behaviors like being rocked as a baby and can help bring the body out of freeze (Ogden et al. 2006).
- Sit in a chair and gently rock back and forth.
- If standing, shift side to side on your feet.
- Imagine rocking yourself to safety.
- If you'd like, you can also combine this rocking with the humming exercise above.

Breath of Fire (Kapalabhati)

The freeze response causes shutdown, numbness and disconnection. Breath of Fire, also known as Kapalabhati, is a cleansing breath practice in yoga that stimulates the diaphragm, vagus nerve and circulation, helping reawaken the body, restore energy and reestablish presence (Sovik 2000). This rhythmic, forceful breathing increases oxygen flow, boosts alertness, raises circulation and bodily presence, counteracts sluggishness, and shifts the nervous system from passive to active (Brown and Gerbarg 2012), activating energy to exit the freeze response.
- Sit or stand comfortably, keeping your spine straight.
- Inhale deeply through your nose, letting your belly expand.

- Exhale forcefully through your nose, pulling your belly in sharply.
- Continue rapid exhales (two or three per second), allowing inhales to happen passively, for thirty seconds to one minute.
- Pause, inhale deeply and exhale slowly.
- Repeat for two or three rounds, adjusting speed if needed.

Anchor Stance

The freeze response can cause the body to collapse inward, creating a curled posture, rounded forward and lacking tone. This is the body's way of conserving energy, but it makes it harder to engage with the world. The anchor stance works as an antidote to freeze by gently activating postural muscles and reestablishing a sense of physical presence. By pressing into the ground and engaging the thighs, you send a signal to your nervous system that it is safe to inhabit your body again.

Although this exercise is especially effective for overcoming the collapsed posture of freeze, it is also helpful for people struggling with the fawn response. Both states involve a loss of personal agency—freeze creates passivity and withdrawal, while fawn results in self-shrinking and excessive compliance. This exercise retrains the body to take up space and feel present in the moment.

- **Stand with your feet hip-width apart.** Visualize your feet sinking into the ground, anchoring you in place. If you are sitting, plant your feet firmly on the floor and imagine them growing heavier.
- **Press your hands firmly against your thighs.** This pressure provides sensory input that helps the nervous system reconnect to the body. Feel the resistance between your hands and thighs—this small engagement can gently pull you out of freeze.
- **Slightly lift your chest and open your shoulders.** Freeze causes the body to curl inward, closing off from

the world. Gently opening the chest helps reverse this withdrawal pattern.
- **Breathe deeply and evenly.** Focus on slow, controlled exhales, which signal safety to the nervous system. As you breathe, repeat internally: *I am here.*
- **Stay in the stance for at least thirty to sixty seconds, or longer if comfortable.** Notice if you feel more engaged, more awake or more connected to your body. If helpful, gently rock your weight from side to side to add a sense of movement without overwhelm.

Regulating the Fawn Response

When the fawn response is activated, we prioritize others' needs at the expense of our own, often suppressing our feelings to avoid conflict or rejection. This can leave us feeling disconnected from ourselves, resentful or emotionally depleted. The goal of fawn-response regulation exercises is to help you reconnect with your own needs, strengthen boundaries and restore a sense of self separate from external approval or performance.

Spoken "No" Practice (Boundary-Setting)

For people stuck in the fawn response, saying no can be difficult. The consequences seem too high and the nervous system associates "no" with danger. Practicing saying no out loud rewires the brain to recognize it as a safe and valid response.
- Find a private space where you feel comfortable speaking out loud.
- Stand or sit in an upright position.
- Take a deep breath and say "No" out loud.
- Experiment with different ways of saying it:
    - Firm: "No."
    - Gentle: "No, thank you."
    - Clear: "That doesn't work for me."

    - Compassionate: "I hear you, but I can't commit to that."
- Repeat five to ten times, noticing how your body feels.
- If any resistance comes up, place a hand on your chest and remind yourself: It is safe for me to have boundaries.

Optional: You can also write out a list of situations you struggle to say no in and practice responding to them in a journal.

Boundary-Setting Through Hands

The fawn response often involves a lack of physical boundaries. Practicing a simple hand gesture reinforces a sense of personal space and teaches your body to stop overextending.
- Stand or sit comfortably.
- Extend both arms in front of you, palms facing forward as if saying "Stop."
- Slowly push outward, feeling your own strength.
- As you do this, internally affirm: I have the right to set boundaries.
- Let your arms return to your sides and notice any shifts in your body.

You can also use props—like pillows, a blanket or a rope—to place a physical boundary around yourself. Experiment with what it feels like to stay within that space and sense others outside of it. Notice what shifts in your body when you give yourself permission to stay centered, rather than crossing that boundary to accommodate someone else.

Everything Out of the Room!

Another aspect of the fawn response is that your nervous system, as a survival response, prioritizes the needs, feelings and expectations of others over your own. Over time, this can make it challenging to know what you truly want, think or feel because your focus is habitually on others. This can result in feeling disconnected from yourself, as if too much of your energy is outside your own body. This is understandable, and we want to help you bring your own energy back to yourself.

This exercise, adapted from our previous book, *Polywise* (2023), is designed to help interrupt the fawn response by removing external influences and reconnecting you with your inner self. By temporarily "clearing the room" of others' opinions, expectations and emotional needs, you create space to be in your own body and fully inhabit yourself. From there, your own desires, preferences and boundaries can emerge more clearly. This practice also gives your nervous system the experience of being safely alone with yourself. For people stuck in the fawn response, alone time doesn't always feel safe—there's often an impulse to check in with others, anticipate their reactions or preemptively adjust to avoid conflict. This practice creates a structured and intentional way to experience a few minutes of solitude in a way that feels grounding, rather than isolating. It gently retrains your body to trust in your own sensations, thoughts and feelings, without having them shaped by the weight of others' needs.

- **Find a private, enclosed space** where you will not be disturbed.
- **Close your eyes** and take a few deep breaths to settle into the present moment. If it helps, imagine letting go of anything from earlier today and temporarily setting aside thoughts about the future.
- **Bring to mind an issue, challenge or decision** during which you have struggled to identify your own perspective.
- **Identify everything that is interfering with your clarity.** Notice whose opinions, expectations or needs are shaping your thoughts. Acknowledge internal pressures such as guilt, obligation or perfectionism. Consider cultural or societal messages that might be influencing you (e.g., "A good partner always prioritizes their relationship" or "It's selfish to put yourself first").

- **Now, put it all out of the room.** One by one, imagine each person stepping outside—partners, family, friends, coworkers. Let go of what you "should" do or how you "should" feel. Place social expectations, guilt, self-judgment and fear outside the room. Only you remain.
- **Breathe into the silence of being alone with yourself.** Notice what it feels like to have only your own energy in the room. Stay with the stillness and let your nervous system register the safety of being with yourself.
- **Now, bring forward the question or situation again.** Ask yourself, either out loud or internally:
  - What is my truth regarding this situation?
  - What are my thoughts? My wants? My feelings? My needs?
  - What do I hope for moving forward?
  - If my opinion or needs mattered just as much as others, what would I do?
- **If external influences try to creep back in,** gently place them back outside.
  - If you notice someone's voice or expectation surfacing, say, "You can wait outside for now."
  - If guilt or obligation arises, remind yourself: This is my time to hear my own voice.
- **When you feel complete, decide what to let back in.** Take a moment to thank everything that stayed outside. Choose what perspectives, if any, you want to consider moving forward.

Listening to the Body's Wisdom

Now that we've explored exercises to regulate your body center, we want to offer a simple practice to listen to this center and connect with its wisdom. Our body holds deep intelligence, and when we learn to listen, it can serve as a compass to guide us.

Settle into Self

Find a comfortable place to sit or lie down. Close your eyes or soften your gaze. Take a few slow, intentional breaths, feeling the weight of your body against the surface beneath you. With each exhale, allow yourself to settle a little more deeply into the present moment. Connect with your Self-energy and abide here for a few moments.

Scan the Body

Bring your attention to your body, scanning from head to toe. Without trying to change anything, simply assess: Where do you feel ease, tension, constriction or numbness? Are there areas that feel heavy, warm, tight or expansive? If certain sensations stand out, stay with them. You are not here to analyze or explain—only to listen.

Ask for the Body's Wisdom

Once you've tuned in, pick a part of your body where you hold tension or an area you are curious about. Choose one sensation that stands out—a tightness in your chest, a heaviness in your stomach, a dull ache in your shoulders or an area that feels disconnected. Without forcing an answer, gently inquire:
- Body, what are you communicating to me here?
- What do you want me to know?
- What do you need?

Receive Without Interference

Let the response arise naturally. It may come as a thought, a feeling, an image or a simple knowing. Or, it may not come right away—that's OK too. Whatever arises, allow it to be there without immediately trying to fix, judge or make sense of it. Your body is offering you wisdom, and your only role is to receive it.

If nothing clear emerges, that's perfectly fine. Simply stay with the sensation, acknowledging its presence and letting it know you are listening. The more often you practice this kind of attention, the more readily your body will share its messages with you.

Bring a Question to Your Body

Now that you've listened and received, you can also bring a question to your body. It can be about anything you are struggling with, a decision you are facing or guidance you need. Instead of thinking through the answer, let your body respond.
- How does this situation feel in my body?
- What direction brings a sense of expansion? What brings constriction?
- What is my body's wisdom on this?

Let your body be a compass, offering direction that may not always make logical sense but is deeply attuned to what you need.

Close with Gratitude

Before finishing, take a moment to thank your body for communicating with you. Even if the message wasn't clear, trust that this connection is strengthening. When you're ready, take a few deep breaths and gently move your body in any way that feels supportive. Carry this awareness forward, knowing that your body is always speaking, always available to be heard.

∆

Your body is more than just a place where the Shame Triangle plays out—it is also where healing begins. It holds deep intelligence. This is why change doesn't come from simply telling yourself you are safe, worthy or enough; your body needs to feel safety, feel connection, feel presence. Those feelings develop through practice: Self-centered practice.

By working with the survival responses covered in this chapter, you've started to lay the groundwork for a different relationship with your body—one where it is not a battleground but a source of wisdom. Just as the Shame Triangle gets wired into our physical responses, the Self-Love Triangle is something we can embody. As we move forward through the Self-centered model, we shift from the body's wisdom to the wisdom of the heart. Many of us have learned to armor our hearts to protect ourselves from pain. And just as we have found ways to regulate and reconnect with the body, we will now explore how to soften the barriers around the heart.

CHAPTER 8
THE SHAME TRIANGLE AND THE HEART

Now, we turn our attention to the heart. As we learned in chapter 5, the heart center can tip into extremes: becoming overactive, overwhelmed by emotion, or underactive, disconnected from feeling altogether. We also examined what a Self-centered heart looks like—one that can hold our feelings, articulate needs and remain open without losing its sense of protection. Before we can access this kind of openness, we must first understand the armor that keeps us guarded and disconnected. The Shame Triangle parts isolate the heart by convincing us that love is not worth it, too dangerous to attempt or unattainable in the first place. If we don't work with this protective layer, the Shame Triangle remains intact, limiting how we give and receive love. Shifting to the Self-Love Triangle isn't just about embracing love—it's about softening the layers of protection that keep us from it.

When open, the heart has an infinite capacity for love—to feel, to connect, to give and receive in ways that are deeply nourishing. This is the best of what it means to have an open heart: to love without fear, to experience intimacy without hesitation. But the heart is also where we carry the weight of our emotional wounds. If love is unreciprocated, when it comes with conditions or when it turns to heartbreak, the heart learns to protect itself. It armors up—not just to block pain, but also to prevent longing that feels unbearable to hold. It's hard to keep the heart open, reaching for love, when that love isn't met in the ways we need or when a relationship we thought was permanent turns into loss. Over time, it can feel easier to close off entirely rather than risk feeling that ache again. Parts of us may decide it's safer to stay distant, to withhold affection or to avoid vulnerability altogether. We convince ourselves that we are unworthy of love or don't really want it. We become emotionally stifled, and in shutting ourselves off, we may avoid the risk of heartbreak, but we also block the very belonging our heart craves.

Although the heart can become guarded, its defenses can also soften. Over time, we can learn to unguard ourselves—not by forcing vulnerability, but by creating enough safety to let the heart open naturally. The key isn't to tear down the armor overnight, but to allow the heart to be both open and protected, rather than walled off or too exposed. When we approach our emotions with Self-energy, the heart becomes an incredible source of wisdom and connection. In this chapter, we share stories of how the heart can open again, and we offer practices to help you connect with your heart, be with your feelings and reshape your heart's armor.

Jessica here!

Throughout my life, I have experienced both significant heartbreaks and heart openings. My earliest heartbreaks stemmed from attachment ruptures: my parents' separation when I was just one year old, my father's absence due to addiction and my beloved stepfather leaving on my seventh birthday. These consequential losses in my formative years left me with an intense longing for connection, but also a guarded approach to romantic love and attachment as I entered adolescence. Growing up poor in Brooklyn, I adopted a tough-girl exterior—a necessary protection that kept me safe, but also kept me distant.

In my twenties, I attended a training where participants were put in groups of three for a heart-opening exercise. One person was the receiver, while the other two offered care. When it was my turn to receive, I lay down while my partners, following the facilitator's guidance, performed a ritual of cleansing my heart. They washed my hands, feet and face with water and rose petals, softly repeating affirmations: "You are safe. You can relax. You are loved." Had I encountered this exercise earlier in life, I would have rolled my eyes and dismissed it. But I was there to learn, and my Inner Coach reminded me that if I wanted change, I needed to try new things, so I fully went with it. By that point in the training, I had already developed a connection with the two givers, which helped me trust in the authenticity of their care.

Overall, it was a beautiful experience, both as the giver and the receiver. But as the receiver, I realized I had never intentionally accepted such tenderness as an adult—at least not outside the context of a romantic relationship, a paid massage or a therapy session. This ritual created space for me to be seen, held and loved in a way I had not been before. Despite being perceived as sweet, friendly and openhearted by those who knew me, I was also highly armored around my heart. I found it easier to give love than to receive it because letting love in would bring me too close to my pain—pain I had deemed strictly off-limits.

Growing up, I developed a strong sense of self-reliance that made it difficult to trust that others could truly support me. I struggled to believe that I could be cared for in a way that met my actual needs rather than serving someone else's agenda. Whenever someone offered genuine support, I craved it, yet I couldn't shake the fear that it might later be used as leverage against me—or that it would be given and then retracted. I wanted to be held, but I didn't trust the hands that reached out. Needless to say, my heart was pretty protected.

This exercise was meant to help me dissolve that armor, but I found it surprisingly difficult to let go. As the guided experience continued, I felt the heaviness in my chest. I saw all the reasons, the memories and the moments that had layered on these completely understandable layers of heart protection. Why on earth would I even consider trying to change it? Then, as I lay there with that question, one of my givers whispered in my ear, "You are so wanted and needed in this world."

That did it! It was exactly what I needed to hear to cut through my defensive layers.

In that moment, my heart exploded open and I felt, all at once, how much I wanted to give. Her words didn't just break through my defenses; they showed me something I had forgotten: that I wasn't just longing to be loved, I was longing to love freely. That's what burst me open. My armor didn't crack because I finally felt worthy of receiving love—it cracked because I finally felt how much I wanted to give it. Tears poured down my face. My givers stayed present, gently wiping my tears as they continued to hold space for me.

At first, the opening in my heart was not relief—it was painful. My chest hurt as I cried. But it wasn't pain from all the love I hadn't received; it was pain from all the love I had held back. The love I had restrained, the care I had withheld. The grief of every moment I had chosen self-protection over connection came rushing out of me. The dam holding my love back broke. But then, beneath it all, something else emerged: a fully intact heart. Even though I had not received the love I needed growing up, my heart still knew how to love. When the armor fell away, my heart didn't have to "figure out" how to love—it simply was love. Without barriers restricting it, love poured out of me, as natural as breathing.

This wasn't the only time my heart cracked open. It has happened again and again—in nature, meditation, falling in love, in parenthood, in deep conversations, reading books, during sex. Each time, my heart opens wider than before, reminding me that while pain and trauma may layer over the process, this breaking is not a shattering—it is an opening.

> But that moment in the training was also not the last time my heart armored itself. Disappointment, breakups, loss, death, embarrassment, regret—all of it continued to impact my heart. These experiences taught me that while love is infinite and the heart is resilient, it is not invincible. People can hurt us, betray us and mishandle our hearts. That is why our hearts should not be given with reckless abandon, especially to those who are unsafe or incapable of caring for them. The key distinction is between habitual armor that blocks the love we want and intentional protection that preserves the love we need.
>
> This is why I make the distinction between armor and a shield. Armor seals us off completely—it's rigid and heavy, and it doesn't allow anything in or out. A shield, on the other hand, is responsive. We can use it when we need it and put it down when we don't. It allows us to move through life with discernment, protecting ourselves without becoming trapped inside our own defenses. Unlike armor, a shield doesn't harden us—it gives us a choice.

If you've been through trauma, the idea of an open heart may seem distant or even impossible. It can feel unfathomable to believe your heart could open again, let alone risk vulnerability with others. That hesitation deserves respect. If this point resonates with you, know that opening your heart does not have to start with another person. It can be a deeply personal journey, a way of reclaiming your inner love—not for someone else, but for yourself. This process is not about forcing connection but about releasing the weight that keeps you from experiencing your own aliveness.

Some people long to open their hearts for the sake of their relationships. Maybe love exists in your life, but you sense its untapped potential. You might feel barriers with people you care about—a yearning for closeness, but an invisible wall in the way. Or perhaps you feel the weight of loneliness even when surrounded by others. If this is the case, your desire to open your heart is a longing to bridge those gaps—to experience the full depth of human connection that you know is possible. By softening the internal barriers around your heart, you can create space for love to flow more freely.

Whether your intention is personal healing or deeper relationships, this journey requires tending. Opening the heart is not a one-time event—it is an ongoing process of allowing and protecting. It requires clearing the armor that no longer serves you while building new, intentional boundaries that do. This interplay between openness and protection is intimately connected to the Shame Triangle. When we believe we are unworthy or unlovable, our Shame Triangle parts tighten the armor around our hearts. My experience in that heart-cleansing ritual showed me that beyond the pain of past wounds, there is often unexpressed love waiting to emerge.

Before we get into exercises, Dave has a story to share too.

David here!

Growing up in a place where violence was prevalent, I was forced to absorb the rules of my environment. While I didn't have the language for it then, I was being taught a rigid script for manhood. From an early age, I understood that toughness was currency, and that masculinity was measured by one's ability to intimidate, to strike first, to never back down. It was all about the way boys spoke to each other, how disputes were settled and where you were in the pecking order. The aggression I experienced was almost always perpetuated by boys who used violence as a means of control and dominance. The most popular kids in my school had physical strength and power over others, which clearly reflected the rules of patriarchy. As a sensitive, thoughtful, creative and introverted child, I could not relate to the expectations of my environment and therefore saw no place for myself in the larger social context. It was confusing, isolating and painful. I felt shame, which only hardened my resolve to protect my heart. This created in me a deep and unconscious mistrust of men that would follow me into my early adulthood. It led to patterns of inner criticism and self-isolation, and I retreated into my intellectual world as a way of escaping the discomfort of my lived experience.

A significant part of that socialization process involved cutting myself off from my feelings of hurt and hiding my emotions—except for anger—because vulnerability equated weakness, and showing it made me an easier target. The unspoken rules of survival dictated that I armor my heart or be seen as prey by those who sought to exploit any perceived weakness. In those moments of anguish and isolation, I longed for connection, for understanding, for a safe space to process the depths of my pain. But the world around me seemed to offer no such sanctuary. Instead, it demanded that I conform to the rigid expectations of masculinity, swallow my emotions and wear a mask of stoicism, lest I be ridiculed or ostracized further. It was a burden that weighed heavily on me and left me feeling disconnected from myself and others.

Despite years of actively working through this early trauma, I continued to struggle with emotional vulnerability, particularly when it came to crying. In relationships, partners would often express difficulty "reading me" or knowing what I was feeling because I wore a mask of practiced indifference and showed no signs of emotion. While I didn't want to be cut off from my emotions, I was—and it was painful to realize I was missing out on the kind of intimacy and connection I genuinely desired. While I had definitely known love in the context of various relationships in my early adulthood—rewarding friendships, caring family members, loving partners—there was a level of commitment and openness that seemed to remain out of reach. What I failed to see then was the way my nervous system was programmed to avoid the depths of emotional intimacy that would actually lead to any kind of secure attachment. It was as if an invisible force field, a barrier erected by my subconscious mind, prevented me from fully surrendering to the vulnerability required for a sustainable connection. The armor that had once protected me now felt like a prison, isolating me from the very thing I desired most: the soul-nourishing intimacy that comes from vulnerability and emotional attunement.

Beneath the layers of armor, I longed for wholeness, for the freedom to love and be loved without reservation. It was a whisper within my being, a call to shed the weight of my past and embrace the present with an open heart. In those moments of clarity, I caught glimpses of the person I could become: unbound by the constraints of fear and trauma, a person who could love deeply and authentically, without the barriers that had once seemed so necessary for survival.

One of the most powerful moments in my life came when my son, Diego, was born. The weeks leading up to his birth were filled with a mix of joyful anticipation and genuine concern. As the due date approached, we learned that he was in the breech position, his little bottom poised to emerge first instead of his head, which threw a monkey wrench into our birthing plan. We were legally no longer able to have a midwife as we had planned, and the doctors warned of the increased risks and likelihood of needing a cesarean delivery. Fortunately, we found the one and only doctor in Denver, Colorado, who would even entertain the idea of Jessica having a vaginal breech birth. However, what had been a mostly smooth pregnancy suddenly escalated into a situation fraught with fear, confronting both of us with the stark realities of life and death.

Leading up to the birth, Jessica tried every technique recommended to coax our son into turning from butt-first to headfirst: spinning on a birthing ball, hot and cold therapy, playing music near her belly, acupuncture, headstands in a pool, Mayan uterine massages, you name it! But Diego seemed determined to enter the world his own way. As the birth began and Jessica's contractions intensified, an undercurrent of fear ran through me. Because Diego was still breech, the hospital room was crowded with more nurses and doctors than usual, creating an atmosphere of heightened tension and anticipation.

What if something went wrong? What if the delivery didn't go smoothly? What if one or both of them died? I had to push those doubts down and be strong for my Jessica, but the pressure of fear persisted.

Witnessing Jessica's process of giving birth—the primal power of it, the unbridled emotion, the strength and absolute vulnerability—was transformative. I had never seen anything like it before. The initial meditative focus she had to keep herself and the baby out of the stress response and then the guttural cries that escaped her lips when contractions picked up. Between contractions, she would describe how it felt like lightning and thunder were striking and rumbling through her body, and like glass was shattering inside her. I already knew she was a powerhouse, but giving birth required both a strength and a surrender in her beyond what either of us ever anticipated. I was witnessing the raw, untamed power of nature itself.

With each contraction, I felt my own breath catch in my throat. Jessica tried to push Diego out, but there wasn't enough movement and the doctors were growing concerned. The atmosphere in the room shifted, becoming more urgent and serious as nurses and doctors prepared for the possibility of surgery. In a last-ditch effort, Jessica changed her position, and suddenly Diego began to emerge. With this adjustment, her efforts finally aligned and Diego was born, transforming the feeling in the room from tense anticipation to overwhelming relief and joy.

In a moment that seemed to stretch into eternity, our baby emerged into the world and I've never felt such relief. All my worries melted away in the face of a process that is both so ordinary and so miraculous. In that moment, I experienced a heart-opening that I will never be able to fully describe. I wept with total abandon, feeling my walls of self-protection completely dismantled through the intensity of it all. The armor that had once seemed so necessary and the emotional barriers I had erected to shield myself from pain crumbled before the sheer force of love and wonder that flooded my being. As I held Diego in my arms, marveling at the perfection of his tiny fingers and the warmth of his skin against mine, I had access to the fullness of my human experience in an entirely new way. It felt incredible. The veil had been lifted, revealing the depths of emotion and connection that I had been denying myself for so long.

The birth of my son cracked that armor wide open and allowed me to finally experience the power of fully embracing vulnerability. As I wept tears of joy, I realized that true strength lies not in denying emotion, but in finding the courage to feel and love wholeheartedly—to love ourselves and others without filters or restrictions. In that sacred moment, I understood that authentic selfhood is defined not by the suppression of emotion, but by the ability to embrace it fully, without apology or reservation. This realization shattered the limiting beliefs about masculinity that had been instilled in me: that to be a "real man" means to be stoic, unemotional, detached. Over time, I learned that being Self-led at the heart center wasn't about forcing my emotions away or pretending I was invulnerable; it meant acknowledging my sadness, fear and longing, while still holding onto a sense of empathy and courage.

It was a rebirth of sorts for me, a shedding of the old skin that had kept me trapped in patterns of disconnection and emotional isolation. As I gazed into the eyes of my newborn son, I made a silent vow to live with an open heart, to model for him the power of vulnerability and the beauty of loving without restraint. That day gave me a vision of walking a new path—one paved with the courage to feel, to connect and to embrace the fullness of my humanity, in all its messy, beautiful and awe-inspiring complexity. It was a transformative realization that forever changed how I viewed myself, my relationships and my role in creating a more just and benevolent world.

These two stories illustrate different paths to opening the heart. For Jessica, this opening occurred during a structured exercise designed to achieve it, while for Dave, it was a spontaneous response to an intense life event. For some, events like birth may be traumatic rather than transformative, and this variability applies to many other life situations as well. Sometimes the bigger experiences of life have enough weight and impact to crack us open, and sometimes the smallest or seemingly most trivial things, like a sappy commercial at just the right moment, are what touch and soften our hearts. We can't always predict what will fortify our defenses or encourage us to shed them. But what we do know is that the state of our heart directly shapes how we relate to others.

It is at this heart center that we most deeply connect to our shared humanity with others. A guarded heart, however, is quick to assume the worst—falling into the Drama Triangle, interpreting others' actions as wrong, off or intentionally harmful. When the heart is closed, we react with defensiveness, suspicion or resentment. But when the heart is open, we are more able to give people the benefit of the doubt, to see their struggles, and to recognize their actions as coming from their own fears, wounds or limitations rather than malicious intent.

This is why cultivating an open heart requires more than just waiting for the right moment. While spontaneous experiences can be powerful, relying solely on them is not enough to sustain a heart that is both open and protected. Whether you experience this shift through a life-changing event, a guided exercise or slow and steady personal growth, the key lies in recognizing that beyond the Shame Triangle–fueled barriers, our hearts naturally lean toward openness and connection.

Reflection Questions

Here are some contemplation questions to explore your own experiences with heart armoring and opening.
- What experiences from your upbringing or past may have contributed to the development of protective armoring around your heart? What fears or hurts led you to guard yourself emotionally? Consider not only major traumas, but also smaller, cumulative experiences.

- What protective behaviors or patterns have you developed over the years in response to these events? How do they show up in your relationships or other areas of life?
- Can you recall times when you found it difficult to receive love, care or nurturing from others? What were the barriers or resistances that arose within you during those moments?
- Reflect on the ways you may have unknowingly withheld your affection, care or compassion from yourself or others out of self-protection. What was the cost of this armoring?
- Have you had any notable heart-opening experiences in your life where you felt a deep sense of connection, vulnerability or unconditional love? What catalyzed that opening, and what did it feel like in your body?
- What have been the smaller or everyday ways your heart has been kept open or not fully closed?
- What practices, relationships or life events have helped soften the armoring around your heart over time? What supports you in being more open and receptive?
- How do you notice your body, heart and mind each responding when your heart begins to close? What cues do you get from each center, and how might focusing on one help you better understand the others?

Heart Center Exercises

Before working on the armor around your heart, it's important to first build the ability to hold your own feelings, to be with your Raw Experience. The following exercises focus on two approaches: externalizing your emotions by seeing them as distinct parts you can engage with and talk to, and turning inward by tuning into your emotions directly and being present with whatever arises.

Both methods help you develop the capacity to be with your feelings, making it easier to soften your heart's defenses. These exercises also help your nervous system learn that it is safe to experience emotions. Once we've practiced this capacity, we'll work on updating your heart's armor and then connect with the luminous, wise heart behind it.

CARE for Your Feelings as Parts

This exercise uses the acronym CARE as a reminder that when we take these steps, we are truly caring for our feelings. This exercise helps you engage with your emotions as separate parts, allowing Self to be with them.

C   Connect with Self

Settle into Self-energy by grounding yourself. Take a few deep breaths and find a sense of steadiness.

A   Allow the Feeling in Front of You

Notice what you're feeling and invite that emotion to step forward as a distinct part. Imagine it externalizing and appearing in front of you at a comfortable distance. Take time to simply allow it to be there. Often, feelings aren't given space or are not used to being with you in Self-energy. Just allowing a feeling to exist in this way can be powerful. Let the externalized part know that you allow it to be here with you right now.

Sometimes, feelings need space to air out, to express themselves fully—whether that means crying, trembling or having a tantrum in front of you. Allow the part to fully embody its emotions as you stay present with it. Your role is to allow and be with it.

R   Receive Its Message

Listen openly. Every part carries a message—it may be holding onto something important, trying to protect you or expressing a need that hasn't been met. Be present with what this part wants to share about its experience. You might ask, "What do you want me to know?" or "What are you trying to point out, protect or take care of?"

As you receive its message, reassure the part that its message makes sense. You might say, "I hear you," "That makes sense" or "I understand why you're here."

Stay with this step until you sense that the part understands that you get it, and it feels recognized and affirmed.

E   Embrace

Offer care in a way that feels natural. You might embrace the part, hold its hand, sit beside it or send out warmth and reassurance from your heart. Let it know it is not alone—you are here with it.

Stay with this step until you sense a shift, no matter how small. The part may settle, relax, soften or take on a different form. Sometimes, a feeling naturally dissolves, transforms into another emotion or moves on entirely. Whatever happens, simply remain present and attuned to what unfolds.

Close the Practice

Thank the part for sharing with you. Gently bring your awareness back to the present moment, feeling your body and breath.

CARE for Your Feelings Inside

This version of CARE focuses on staying with your emotions internally, rather than externalizing them as parts. Instead of imagining the feeling outside of you, allow it to exist fully within you—wherever it shows up in your body. You are staying blended with the feeling while still accessing Self-energy. The goal is to make space for the feeling inside you, allowing it to be there without resistance, suppression or the need to change.

C   Connect with Self

Settle into Self-energy by grounding yourself. Take a few deep breaths and find a sense of inner stillness. Feel your body and the support beneath you.

A   Allow the Feeling Within

Pick a feeling you want to work with, or decide to work with a feeling that is already present. Turn your attention inward and notice where the feeling is located in your body. Bring your awareness to it. Give it permission to exist exactly as it is. Sometimes, emotions feel stuck because they've never been given space to simply be.

If the feeling needs to expand, contract, pulse, vibrate or move, let it. Stay with it and allow it to unfold in its own way. If it begins to feel overwhelming, gently reassure it: "I'm here now. You don't have to overwhelm me to get my attention." This simple acknowledgment helps the feeling settle, knowing it's being heard.

R   Receive Its Message

Instead of analyzing or explaining the feeling from your mind center, listen from your heart center to what it wants to communicate. Every emotion carries meaning—it might be trying to tell you something about your needs, past experiences or something unresolved. You can ask, "What are you trying to show me?", "What do you want me to know?" or "What are you protecting or holding for me?"

As you receive its message, reassure the feeling that it makes sense. You might say, "I hear you," "That makes sense" or "I understand why you're here."

Stay with this step until the feeling seems understood and validated.

E   Embrace

Now, from Self, extend care and warmth from within. You might place a hand over the area where you feel the feeling most, breathe into it or simply hold it in your awareness with openness.

Stay in this embrace until you sense some kind of shift—even a slight settling, loosening or change in sensation. Sometimes, emotions dissolve, transform or move through naturally once they are fully allowed. Whatever happens, remain present with what unfolds.

Close the Practice

Gently bring your awareness back to your breath and the present moment. Feel your body, your surroundings and the space you are in. Acknowledge yourself for staying with the feelings that arose.

Releasing the Weight of the Heart

After caring for your feelings, you may need to do more than just witness their pain, hurt or emotional burdens—you may need to help release them. When a part or feeling has been seen and allowed, it may reach a point where it's ready to let go of what it's been holding. This practice can be used in conjunction with the CARE methods above, whenever a part is ready to move from being held to being unburdened.

When you sense that a part or feeling is ready to release something, ask for clear confirmation. If it's ready, invite it to show you how it would like to let go of what it's been carrying. It may want to send the pain down a river, burn it in a fire, bury it deep in the earth, cast it into the wind or hand it off to a trusted presence. It can also be helpful to visualize the burden coming out the bottom of your body and releasing into the ground, letting the earth receive and transform it. Let the part choose the method that feels most natural, trusting that the elements—earth, water, fire, air—can help transform and carry away what no longer serves.

Stay with the release as it happens. Notice any physical or emotional shifts. Let whatever comes be part of the process. Once the burden has been released, ask the part what it would like to receive in place of the burden. It might choose certain qualities or strengths to embrace. Allow that energy to move into the space that's been cleared. To close this practice, thank the part for its willingness to let go. Take a few breaths. Feel your body, your heart and the space you've created.

(For more ways to release burdens, the following two chapters offer several alternative practices you can explore.)

Updating Your Heart's Protection

This exercise helps you identify and update the emotional armor around your heart, replacing rigid, outdated defenses with a more flexible, responsive form of protection. The goal is not to remove your armor entirely, but to shift it into something adaptable—more like a shield than a wall—so that you can balance openness with safety. Your armor is a protector, much like the parts in your Shame Triangle, and it deserves to be acknowledged, rather than forced away.

When you tune into yourself and sense the armor around your heart, it may be a Shame Triangle part that has taken on a protective role, or it might be an entirely separate part with its own purpose. Many people experience their heart protection as a physical barrier—a wall, a cage, barbed wire or metallic plating—but whatever form it takes, you can externalize it and engage with it.

Connect to Self

Take a few deep breaths and settle into Self-energy. Feel the support beneath you and center yourself in the present moment.

Tune In to the Heart and Identify Your Armor

Bring your awareness to your heart area. Invite any armoring to reveal itself, whether as a part, image, sensation, thought or memory. Stay open and curious. What does your armor look like? How does it feel?
- Does it come from a Shame Triangle part, such as your Inner Critic, Escaper or Shame itself?
- Is it something distinct or separate from these parts?
- What is its texture, weight or shape? Does it feel solid, heavy or restrictive?

Dialogue with Your Armor

Once you've identified the armor, engage with it as a part. How did it come to be? What is its role? What does it believe it's protecting you from? How has it helped you in the past?

You already know this armor is here to protect you. Appreciate it for the role it has played—it developed for a reason, often in response to situations where your heart was vulnerable. Let it know that you are no longer in those original conditions and that, while protection is still needed, it can be more adaptable now.

Explain to this protector that although it has done its job well, it has also been overprotective, making it harder for love, care and affection to flow in and out. Ask if it would be willing to shift into a form that allows you to stay protected, but also connected.

Reshape Your Protection

Talk with your armor about how it might take on a new, more flexible form. Here are some examples of how people have shifted their armor:
- A solid metal suit enclosing the heart became a samurai standing guard beside it.
- A stone wall transformed into a protective home with doors and windows that can open as needed.

- A locked gate became a drawbridge that can be raised or lowered depending on what's needed.
- A guard dog that barked at everything became a loyal companion—alert and protective, but able to tell the difference between real danger and a passing noise.
- A suit of armor, a thick shell or a heavy barricade transformed into a shield—something that can be used to deflect and protect when needed, but can also be set down when it's not.

What new form of protection would feel right for you? Let your armor adjust and evolve into something that supports both your safety and your ability to love freely.

Install Your New Protection

Visualize this new, responsive form of protection fully taking shape. Introduce it to your heart and clearly communicate how you would like it to function.
- How should it protect you?
- How should it be discerning and alert you to real threats without blocking connection unnecessarily?

Close the Practice

Take a few moments to thank this new protector for working with you. Gently bring your awareness back to your breath and your body. Move slowly, stretch if needed and acknowledge yourself for taking the time to work through your heart's protection.

Consider journaling about the new protective measures you've installed and any insights you gained from the exercise. To reinforce the shift, tune in to this updated protector on a regular basis, reminding your heart and its protection of their new role.

Luminous Heart Meditation

This meditation helps awaken your heart's innate capacity for love, using the imagery of a radiant, ever-expanding sun within you.

Sit or lie down in a comfortable, quiet space where you won't be disturbed.

Ground and center yourself. Close your eyes and begin to focus on your breath. Inhale deeply through your nose, hold for a few seconds and exhale slowly through your mouth. Settle into Self-energy. Unblend from any parts if needed.

Visualize your heart as a sun. Imagine a radiant sun within your chest, pulsing with warm, golden light. This is a source of infinite love and compassion.

With each inhale, expand the light. Visualize this sun growing brighter and more luminous. As you exhale, allow its warmth to spread throughout your body, melting any tension or resistance it encounters. Take time to enjoy this step.

Visualize the rays of your heart sun extending beyond your body, filling the room and beyond with its healing light. Just as the sun is the source of light, feel yourself as a source of radiating love.

Silently repeat an affirmation that resonates with this radiant heart energy, such as "My heart is open. My heart shines brightly. I am Love. I radiate love to myself and others."

Give and receive love. Imagine yourself both basking in and emanating this warm, loving light. Allow yourself to receive this love fully, and then consciously send it out to others.

Close the practice. When you're ready, slowly bring your awareness back to your physical surroundings. Take a moment to appreciate the warmth and openness in your heart before opening your eyes.

Connecting with Your Wise Heart

This exercise connects you with the wisdom of your Self-centered heart.

Sit or lie down in a comfortable, quiet place where you won't be disturbed.

Ground and center in Self. Close your eyes and focus on your breath. Inhale deeply through your nose, hold for a few seconds and exhale slowly through your mouth. Repeat several times, allowing yourself to settle and tune in to Self-energy.

Visualize your awakened heart. Imagine it as a radiant sun, a fully bloomed flower or a wise and loving presence. This is your heart in its most open and awakened state—full of love, wisdom and clarity. Stay here for a moment and simply be with your heart, feeling its fullness. If you sense any heart protection, gently ask it to step aside for this exercise.

Connect with your awakened heart. With each breath, feel yourself in conversation with your heart. What does it embody? How does it communicate with you? You can ask for guidance, pose a question or simply listen. Allow your heart's wisdom to flow freely to you. Listen and be with it.

Step into or merge with the presence of your fully awakened heart. Feel its qualities—unconditional love, wisdom, strength and deep knowing—becoming part of you.

Radiate love. From this place of embodiment, visualize love and compassion flowing from your heart, expanding outward to others and the world.

Close the practice. Thank your wise heart for its presence and guidance. Slowly bring your awareness back to your physical surroundings, carrying this connection with you. When you're ready, gently open your eyes.

Δ

The heart is the most courageous part of us—not because it never fears, but because it continues to love despite fear. It opens, even after hurt. It longs, even when longing has led to disappointment. The challenge is not that we feel too much; the challenge is that we were never taught how to hold what we feel with care.

In this chapter, we explored how the Shame Triangle isolates the heart—how it convinces us that love is dangerous, that we are too much or not enough, that we must either protect ourselves at all costs or abandon ourselves entirely. But when the heart is Self-centered, it does not collapse under its emotions, nor does it harden itself against them. It learns to hold both joy and pain, connection and loss, belonging and solitude.

As we move forward, we turn our attention to the mind—the meaning-maker. If the body is where we store our experiences and the heart is where we feel them, the mind is where we make sense of them. It is also where the Shame Triangle holds some of its deepest strongholds—old beliefs, rigid thinking and narratives that convince us that nothing can change. But just as the body can be rewired and the heart can be softened, the mind can be reshaped into an ally, rather than an adversary.

CHAPTER 9
THE SHAME TRIANGLE AND THE MIND

The Shame Triangle obviously influences how we think about ourselves. It takes hold of the mind more powerfully than almost anything else. In the mind center, the Shame Triangle shows up as rigid, absolute beliefs—many of them harsh and unquestioned—that convince us they are facts rather than learned patterns that can be changed. Confronting these beliefs is one of the greatest challenges in healing. Even if you've already felt shifts in your Shame Triangle parts, the familiar pull of self-deprecating narratives can make it easy to slip back into old thought patterns, reinforcing the illusion that they are true. Returning to these thought patterns can lead to discouragement, or even to abandoning the process of working to transform your Shame Triangle altogether. After years, sometimes a lifetime, of believing something is fundamentally wrong with you or that you must change to be loved and accepted, shifting your mindset requires intentional support.

The mind can be like a well-worn path. If you've walked the same route every day, it's easy to forget that other ways exist. But the mind is also pliant. It can be reshaped, rewired and restored. A Self-centered mind is one that can recognize these ingrained beliefs, question them and create space for new perspectives. By working with these Shame Triangle mindsets, we begin to untangle ourselves from them and reclaim the mind as a place of clarity and insight. In this chapter, we'll break down the mindsets most closely tied to the Shame Triangle, explore their antidotes and offer exercises for working with difficult beliefs.

Shame Triangle Mindsets

The Adversarial Mindset

The adversarial mindset operates on a "me versus you" or "us versus them" framework, positioning people as opponents, rather than allies. In this mindset, conflict is seen as a battle to win, not a problem to solve, and differences between people are treated as threats, rather than opportunities. From an early age, we are taught, whether explicitly or implicitly, that life is about proving ourselves against others. In school, we are graded on a curve, ranked against our peers and measured by how we compare. In sports, even in team-based games where cooperation is essential, the focus is still on winning and losing—reinforcing the idea that our success comes at someone else's expense. Social media amplifies this mindset, turning visibility into a competition for likes, followers and engagement, where attention feels like something to win rather than something to share.

We see the adversarial mindset in a justice system that prioritizes punishment over resolution, in entertainment that thrives on rivalries, and in political news that reduces complex issues to battles between heroes and villains. It even shapes how we interact with strangers. If someone cuts us off in traffic, we assume they're selfish or reckless, rather than considering they might be rushing to a hospital. If a coworker doesn't acknowledge us in the hallway, we take it as a slight, rather than recognizing that they might be lost in thought or having a hard day. The adversarial mindset leads us to assume hostility where there may be none. This way of thinking might seem justified in an unfair world filled with real dangers, identity theft and increasingly elaborate scams. But when we project it everywhere, we lose our ability to see what a more collaborative, non-adversarial stance can offer.

Even in our closest relationships, we can forget that we're on the same team. Instead, we posture against each other, treating conflicts as battles to prove who is right. Loved ones become opponents and disagreements feel like contests to be won, rather than opportunities for understanding. Rather than reaching for connection, we armor up, convinced we must protect ourselves from being wronged, exposed or hurt. When we internalize this mindset, it turns both our inner and outer worlds into minefields. We approach our mistakes as failures. We hear feedback as an attack. We brace ourselves for criticism, as if one wrong move could cost us our dignity, relationships or success. This state of hypervigilance and defensiveness creates the perfect conditions for the Shame Triangle to take hold, making us adversaries within ourselves.

Reflection Questions

- In what areas of your life does adversarial thinking (e.g., defensiveness, competitiveness, "me versus you" thinking) show up most prominently?
- Where have you experienced adversarial thinking from others, and what impact has that had on you?
- Consider each part of your Shame Triangle. Which parts exhibit an adversarial mindset? How does it manifest, and what are its effects on your thoughts, emotions and behaviors?
- In what ways has the adversarial mindset been reinforced in your life through family dynamics, education, work environments or societal messages?

- How has the adversarial mindset affected your relationships, both personal and professional? Can you identify any patterns or recurring issues?

The Binary Mindset

While the adversarial mindset pits "us" against "them," binary thinking flattens our experience of life into rigid either/or categories. It forces us to see the world in black and white—right or wrong, success or failure, lovable or unlovable—stripping away the vast spectrum of possibilities that truly exist. This kind of thinking appears everywhere. It tells us that people must fit neatly into one of two boxes: male or female, Democrat or Republican, good or bad, straight or gay, success or failure. It reduces intelligence to smart or dumb, attractiveness to pretty or ugly, strength to powerful or weak, and personal value to worthy or unworthy. But life doesn't work that way. These binaries often represent only the endpoints of a broad, rich spectrum, flattening all the middle ground in between. People are complex, identities are layered and circumstances are fluid. We don't always fall at one end of a spectrum—often we're somewhere in between, exactly where we belong, even if that doesn't fit the binary. No one is just one thing. Yet binary thinking erases nuance, making it easy to judge ourselves and others without considering the full picture.

When we apply the rigid framework of the binary mindset to ourselves, it solidifies our Shame Triangle. Every perceived flaw or shortcoming becomes proof that we belong in a "bad" category. If we don't feel "good enough" in some area of life, the only alternative seems to be that we're a total failure—rather than recognizing that we're simply in the process of learning and growing, or that we're in the messy, competent, very human middle. When a relationship hits a rough patch, this mindset tells us we're either built for love or doomed to be alone. When we stumble in a new skill or get passed over for a promotion, it convinces us we're fundamentally unfit, instead of seeing a temporary setback for what it is. Binary thinking denies the legitimacy of middle-ground experiences—of being OK, capable or comfortable in places that don't fit tidy labels or extremes. This kind of thinking leaves no room for being imperfect, real humans who are steady and content with who and where and how we are.

Reflection Questions

- In what areas of your life does binary thinking (e.g., all or nothing, success or failure, right or wrong) show up most prominently?
- Where have you observed binary thinking in others, and what impact has that had on you?
- Consider each part of your Shame Triangle. Which parts rely on a black-and-white approach? How does this mindset influence your thoughts, emotions and behaviors?
- How do you perceive internal conflict with your different parts? Do you tend to see them as opponents or allies?
- In what ways has binary thinking been reinforced in your life (through family dynamics, education, workplace culture or societal norms)?
- How has an either/or mindset affected your relationships, both personal and professional? Can you identify any recurring patterns or issues?

The Fixed Mindset

Stanford psychologist Carol Dweck became curious when she noticed that some university students who failed or performed poorly responded with resilience, while others shut down entirely. Through her research, Dweck discovered that the difference between the two groups wasn't their intelligence or ability—it was their *beliefs* about their intelligence and ability. Students who thought their skills were fixed—who believed they were simply "bad at math" or "not smart enough"—became trapped in cycles of self-doubt and poor performance. Meanwhile, those who saw intelligence as something that could grow with effort continued to improve. Dweck coined the term "fixed mindset" to describe the belief that intelligence, talents and abilities are set in stone (2006). This mindset is reflected in phrases like, "You either have it or you don't," "Some people are just naturally gifted" or "I'll never be able to do that." It convinces us that our abilities or worth are predetermined, leaving little room for growth.

This viewpoint sees skills as static rather than malleable, so every stumble or shortcoming is interpreted as a permanent reflection of who we are, not just a bump in the road. This way of thinking shows up in everyday life more than we realize. Sayings like "You can't teach an old dog new tricks," "That's just who I am" or "I'm too old for this" all reinforce the idea that change isn't possible. This mindset also appears when people treat their astrological sign, personality type or attachment style as an unshakable identity, rather than a collection of tendencies that can shift and evolve. A fixed mindset locks preferences, habits and perceived traits into rigid categories, shaping our behaviors in ways that reinforce limitation rather than possibility.

This is the Shame Triangle's natural habitat. Some parts believe change is hopeless and resign themselves to self-defeat. Others latch onto the idea that we *can* change—but only by force, only by being *fixed*. Not through curiosity, not through growth, but through persistent inner policing and the hope that if we just work hard enough, we'll finally be acceptable. In both cases, the outcome is the same: The mind stays fixed.

Reflection Questions

- In which areas of your life do you tend to believe that your abilities or traits are "set in stone"?
- How have these beliefs been reinforced by others or by your environment? Consider messages you've heard at

home, in school, at work or in society that encouraged you to think you "are" a certain way—smart, lazy, responsible—and can't deviate from it.
- Look at each part of your Shame Triangle. Where do you notice a fixed mindset?
- How do you typically react when you face setbacks or challenges? Where in your life does a fixed mindset most powerfully influence your response?
- What effects does a fixed mindset have on your relationships?

The Expert Mindset

The expert mindset is the belief that our knowledge or perspective is inherently superior to that of others. It comes with an unshakable sense of certainty—"Father knows best" or "Don't question me, I'm the authority." When in this mindset, we position ourselves above those around us, convinced that we know more—even about their own experiences. This isn't just confidence or strong self-esteem; it's the rigid belief that our understanding is not only greater, but makes us better. At its core, this is a "power over" stance, one that can become dangerous, whether we use our perceived expertise to control others or, conversely, surrender our power to those deemed "experts."

When the expert mindset spills over into relationships, it often shows up as monologuing rather than genuine dialogue, focusing on proving one's point instead of truly listening, or playing devil's advocate rather than asking genuine questions. When in this mindset, we tend to prioritize being "smart" or "right" above all else, believing that any deviation from certainty reveals weakness. As a result, differing views or people with information beyond our expertise can feel like a threat to our sense of self, causing us to retreat or double down on our position. The irony is that by insisting we already "know," we miss out on valuable opportunities to learn from others and stifle our chance to actually increase our expertise on something by staying open, curious and willing to be changed by what we hear.

> **Reflection Questions**

- Where in your life do you tend to adopt an "expert" position? Think of situations—whether at work, in your family or among friends—where you feel certain you "know best" or have superior knowledge.
- How have you experienced the expert mindset from others, and what impact did it have on you? Reflect on times when someone else's certainty or know-it-all attitude made you feel unheard, dismissed or undermined in your own perspective.
- Consider each part of your Shame Triangle. Which part, if any, might exhibit an expert mindset?
- In what ways has the expert mindset been reinforced in your life? Examine the family dynamics, educational settings, work environments or societal messages that may have encouraged or rewarded a "power over" stance.
- How has this mindset shaped your relationships, both personal and professional? Can you identify any patterns, such as arguing instead of listening, or dismissing others' perspectives? Where might curiosity and openness enhance these connections?

Self-Led Mindsets

When we're locked into a certain mindset, it can be difficult to recognize. We become like a radio stuck on a single station, unaware that countless other frequencies exist. Then, a new perspective appears—like a doorway to fresh possibility—and suddenly the beliefs that once felt solid begin to show their cracks. Seeing these limitations can sharpen our sense of what truly matters and spark a desire for change. But even with this clarity, shifting our thinking isn't always straightforward. The same problem-saturated thought loops that kept us stuck often try to pull us back in.

That's because we're not just tweaking surface-level ideas—we're talking about deeper shifts in how we perceive and experience life. And while the insight may come quickly, integration rarely does. Even after exposing the distortions of the Shame Triangle, it's common to slip back under their spell. For many of us, fully embodying new beliefs is neither quick nor easy. We may feel internal resistance as we begin to detox from the inherited mindsets shaped by family, culture and dominant social narratives. Sometimes, it feels as though we're trying to let go of beliefs that don't want to let go of us, making it difficult to stabilize new ways of thinking, even when we're ready for them.

Thankfully, the good news is that simply being exposed to new mindsets can have a psychoactive effect. Like a flash of light in a dark room, they can illuminate patterns we didn't even know we were trapped in. Even a brief encounter with a new way of thinking can disrupt old loops, stretch our mental boundaries and spark a sense of possibility that's hard to unsee. The practice then becomes initiating the shift—and returning to it, again and again—until it begins to stabilize as the mind's new default. As we move beyond the limiting frameworks that fuel the Shame Triangle, we're not just swapping one set of beliefs for another; we're stepping into entirely new paradigms that transform how we relate to ourselves and others. Below are four powerful mindset shifts that help move us from the constricting beliefs of the Shame Triangle to the expansive perspectives of the Self-Love Triangle.

- **From Adversarial Paradigm to Restorative Paradigm:** Shift from viewing people as adversaries and conflict as a battle to be won toward seeing conflict as an opportunity for empathy, collaboration and genuine connection.
- **From Binary Thinking to Non-Dual Consciousness:** Move beyond rigid either/or extremes to embrace a

broader spectrum of possibilities and perspectives, fostering a more holistic and inclusive worldview.
- **From Fixed Mindset to Growth Mindset:** Replace the belief that abilities are set in stone with the understanding that challenges fuel learning and evolution, recognizing effort and perseverance over innate talent.
- **From Expert Mindset to Beginner's Mindset:** Let go of the need to be "right" or in control and instead adopt curiosity, embrace not knowing and value the discovery process over appearing knowledgeable.

By adopting these Self-Love Triangle antidotes, we can more effectively deconstruct the limiting beliefs that underpin the Shame Triangle and resist their influence, while at the same time begin to integrate ways of thinking that will continue to strengthen our connection to genuine Self-energy.

These are some of the key shifts from limiting mindsets to more expansive, restorative ways of thinking, including some of the qualities or values that these mindsets focus on or embrace.

Limiting Mindset		Expansive Mindset
Adversarial		**Restorative**
Competition	→	Collaboration
Judgment	→	Understanding
Blame	→	Accountability
Division	→	Connection
Punishment	→	Repair
Binary Thinking		**Non-Dual**
Either/Or	→	Both/And
Separation	→	Interconnection
Absolutes	→	Complexity
Rigidity	→	Flexibility
Opposition	→	Integration

Fixed		**Growth**
Limitation	→	Possibility
Failure	→	Learning
Stagnation	→	Adaptability
Avoiding Challenges	→	Embracing Challenges
Innate Talent	→	Effort and Progress
Expert		**Beginner's**
Certainty	→	Curiosity
Proving	→	Learning
Defending	→	Exploring
Control	→	Openness
Knowing	→	Discovering

The Restorative Mindset

If the Adversarial Mindset sees life as a battlefield—where others are opponents and survival means defeating someone else—the Restorative Mindset is more like a thriving forest. In a forest, every plant, animal and fungus plays a role in maintaining the health of the whole ecosystem. Instead of competition, there's interdependence: a web of support that allows everything to flourish. The restorative mindset is built on collaboration, empathy and shared humanity. It recognizes that we are all connected and reframes differences, misunderstandings and conflict as opportunities to come closer, rather than grow apart. Instead of pitting people against each other, it asks: How can we repair, learn and move forward together?

This approach isn't new. It has long been a part of the traditions and philosophies of many Indigenous cultures worldwide. Our perspective on the restorative mindset is shaped by restorative justice, a movement that emerged in the United States in the 1970s in response to the failures of traditional, punishment-based systems. Reform advocates like Howard Zehr (1990) recognized that simply handing down sentences or imposing criminal records often did more harm than good, especially to society's most vulnerable people. In contrast, restorative justice focuses on accountability, healing and community support. Its principles draw from Indigenous traditions such as Navajo Peacemaking and First Nations circle processes, which emphasize repairing relationships rather than punishing wrongdoing.

Both of us have trained as restorative justice facilitators, and we've seen firsthand how these practices offer an alternative to the typical punitive approach. For example, if a teenager is caught shoplifting, instead of facing juvenile detention, they would be invited to meet with the person or business they harmed, acknowledge the impact of their actions and work toward making amends. Community members also take part, ensuring that accountability is paired with support and fairness for everyone involved. Building on these principles, Dave later developed the Restorative Relationship Conversations model, applying restorative justice to intimate relationships to help loved ones repair conflict and harm between them. We've seen time and again how shifting from an adversarial, Drama and Shame Triangle–driven stance to a Self-led, restorative Self-Love Triangle approach transforms conflicts that once felt hopeless. By focusing on repair instead of blame and connection instead of division, people heal long-standing wounds and rebuild trust in ways they never thought possible.

Just as a restorative approach can repair external conflict, it can reshape how we relate to ourselves. Within the Shame Triangle, we often fall into patterns of blame, shutdown or avoidance. A restorative mindset helps us see what each part is trying to communicate or protect. When that purpose is recognized, the internal friction begins to settle. Our parts become more responsive, more willing to engage and more able to work together. Over time, this approach creates a new internal culture—a culture of collaboration, not conflict—where understanding takes precedence over judgment. (Chapter 11 walks you through a step-by-step process for applying restorative principles to your Shame Triangle parts.)

The Non-Dual Mindset

Binary thinking reduces life to "all or nothing," leaving little room for the complexity of our real lived experiences. The non-dual mindset is a psychological, philosophical and spiritual perspective that offers a different way of seeing the world—one that moves beyond rigid categories and embraces the full spectrum of reality. Strength and vulnerability, logic and emotion, mind and body, love and resentment, success and failure—these are not irreconcilable opposites but interconnected aspects of a greater whole. Rather than choosing one or the other, the non-dual mindset invites us to hold two or more truths at once—even when they seem at odds. Instead of dividing everything into right or wrong, good or bad, this or that, non-dual awareness helps us accept a wider range of truth and experience.

Rather than forcing either/or choices, the non-dual mindset invites both/and thinking. You can feel frustrated, grateful and unsure all at once in a relationship with a friend. You can believe in yourself and still experience self-doubt. A painful ending can also mark the beginning of something meaningful. This mindset helps us stay in the gray space—not just between two poles, but in the full range of feeling, perception and experience—where life is most honest, nuanced and alive, and where multiple truths can coexist.

Each Shame Triangle part is trapped in binary thinking, but when Self engages from a broader, more nuanced perspective, it introduces flexibility and understanding. We can acknowledge the Inner Critic's protective intent while recognizing that its harshness is harmful. We can see the Escaper's instinct to avoid pain as natural, while also knowing that real relief comes from facing discomfort, not fleeing from it.

A non-dual mindset dissolves the rigid logic that keeps the Shame Triangle in place. It allows us to hold conflicting truths at once—we can be independent *and* in need of help, strong *and* vulnerable. We can be falling apart *and* still have our shit together. Our experiences, emotions and identities exist on a spectrum, not in defined categories. By releasing binary thinking, we step into the Self-Love Triangle, where we can see ourselves and our experiences with greater clarity, making space for complexity, contradiction and coexistence. This shift allows us to respond to life with more discernment and adaptability, rather than rigid, all-or-nothing thinking.

The Growth Mindset

In her research on the fixed mindset, psychologist Carol Dweck found that people who believed their abilities, intelligence and potential were unchangeable tended to avoid challenges, give up easily and see effort as a sign of inadequacy. In contrast, those who saw abilities as something that could develop with time and practice—who displayed what Dweck called a growth mindset— were more likely to embrace challenges, persist through setbacks and ultimately improve. In *Mindset: The New Psychology of Success* (2006), Dweck emphasized that adopting a growth mindset isn't about blind optimism or forcing positivity. It requires actively questioning self-limiting beliefs, seeing mistakes as information rather than failure, and understanding that progress is built through effort, not innate ability.

This shift is critical when moving from the Shame Triangle's rigid, self-defeating beliefs to the flexibility of a Self-centered mind. A fixed mindset keeps us trapped, making struggles feel like proof that we are flawed or incapable. When we fail at something, we assume it's because we're just bad at it, rather than recognizing that failure is part of any learning process. The growth mindset challenges this belief by disrupting the Shame Triangle's certainty that we *are* our limitations. It shifts the focus from "I can't" to "I haven't yet," from self-condemnation to self-discovery. Instead of seeing setbacks as confirmations of unworthiness, we begin to see them as stepping stones toward deeper understanding, skill-building and resilience. This change isn't instant or easy. It requires consistent practice, but over time it rewires how we relate to difficulty and self-doubt.

Yet growth isn't always about changing our circumstances. Some aspects of ourselves, or our lives, may not be within our control. But while we may not always be able to change our situation, we can always change how we relate to it. The growth mindset helps us shift from resistance to agency, from helplessness to adaptability, from being a victim to a conscious participant. It allows us to approach even the unchangeable with curiosity, creativity and a sense of possibility, rather than feeling stuck in resignation. Even when life presents real limitations, we can choose whether we see them as walls that trap us or landscapes we learn to navigate.

The Beginner's Mindset

While the growth mindset focuses on believing in our capacity to improve through effort, the beginner's mindset is about how we approach life itself—with openness, curiosity and a willingness to experience things as they are. True wisdom doesn't come from certainty but from staying open to the unknown. The beginner's mindset comes from the Zen Buddhist concept of Shoshin, which means approaching life with a fresh perspective, free from rigid assumptions, no matter how much experience or knowledge we have. Zen master Shunryu Suzuki, in *Zen Mind, Beginner's Mind* (1970), famously wrote, "In the beginner's mind there are many possibilities, but in the expert's mind there are few." When we are new to something, we naturally approach it with curiosity. We ask questions, explore possibilities and remain flexible in our thinking. But as we gain knowledge or expertise, we often close down, assuming we already know enough. We can become more invested in proving what we know rather than discovering what we don't.

This contrast is what makes the beginner's mindset so transformative. The expert mindset thrives on certainty and the need to be right, while the beginner's mindset embraces the reality that we never fully know everything. While we can have moments of confidence, true understanding requires staying open, continuing to learn and letting go of rigid conclusions. The expert mind seeks validation, resists uncertainty and fears looking foolish, while the beginner's mind values learning, exploration and being fully present with what is. Instead of clinging to what we already know, it allows us to see the world and ourselves with fresh eyes.

A common struggle many people experience is jumping to negative conclusions, especially in moments of uncertainty. Take, for example, waiting for a response to a text. Instead of assuming the delay is neutral, the mind often leaps to the worst possible interpretation: *They're ignoring me. They don't care. I must have done something wrong.* Anxious thoughts spiral, worst-case scenarios take over, and sometimes people even send reactive messages before the other person has had a chance to reply. This is a mind stuck in certainty—that something bad has happened, that they are being ghosted, that they are at fault. But this certainty is based on stories the mind is spinning, not fact.

A beginner's mindset in this scenario would allow for a different response. Instead of fixating on a single negative explanation, it would stay open to multiple possibilities: *Maybe they're caught up at work. Maybe they're having a hard day. Maybe their phone is off or they typed a response but accidentally didn't hit send.* When we acknowledge multiple possibilities, we stop filling in the blanks with a negative two-dimensional, typically self-focused story and instead allow a more open-ended, "I don't know" stance—which, ironically, is usually much closer to the truth.

The same principle applies to the Shame Triangle. Each part clings to rigid conclusions about who we are, how others see us or what a particular emotion must mean. But these conclusions are just interpretations shaped by past experiences—not truths carved in stone. When Self leads with a beginner's mindset, we create room to ask different questions. We don't shut down or rush to fix what we're feeling. We wonder. We explore. We ask: What else might be true here? What have I not considered?

The beginner's mindset teaches us that not knowing is not a weakness—it's where growth begins. Yet many people fear looking inexperienced or making mistakes, as if competence should come instantly and being a beginner is something to be embarrassed about. People then hesitate to ask questions, admit gaps in knowledge or struggle through new experiences because they fear looking incompetent. But the beginner's mindset frees us from the pressure to perform, impress or be right. Instead, we get to engage with life as it unfolds: learning, adjusting, stumbling, laughing and growing.

Shift Your Mindset Prompts

The work in this book is already helping you access and cultivate these Self-centered mindsets. Being in Self brings you closer to them, and the more you practice leading from Self, the more these perspectives will become second nature. The more we strengthen our ability to pause and shift perspectives, the easier it becomes to step out of problem-saturated mindsets. What's powerful about these shifts is that simply being exposed to different ways of thinking creates choice in places where it previously felt like there was none. Just knowing that alternative perspectives exist opens new ways of seeing that weren't available before, creating a path out of habitual ways of thinking. Because of this benefit, we've found that using specific prompts to access a more Self-led mindset can actually create the shift itself. The moment we consider a new possibility, we pivot from the old mindset and step into something wider, freer and more relational.

To support this process, we offer specific prompts designed to interrupt old patterns and guide you toward a more Self-led, open perspective. A well-known example of this kind of shift comes from couples therapy. When working with partners in conflict, especially when one is fixated on proving their point and being right about the "facts" of what happened, a therapist might ask, "Do you want to be right, or do you want to be in relationship?" This question isn't about dismissing truth or stamping out valid concerns; it's about shifting focus. It moves a person from an adversarial or expert stance—where proving a point is the priority—into a more relational, restorative mindset, where understanding and connection take center stage.

When someone is locked in the need to be right, they often feel compelled to prove their point, establish facts or demonstrate that they remember events exactly as they happened. Yet this approach rarely persuades the other person and often leads to more defensiveness and disconnection. But when the focus shifts from being right to being in relationship, defenses lower and hearts soften. This shift applies to our inner world as well.

While the prompts that follow are written in a "this or that" format, they are not about labeling one side as good and the other as bad. Their purpose is to loosen the grip of reactive mindsets and open a doorway into a more Self-led, spacious way of relating. The irony is that what might appear like a binary is actually a bridge. Each prompt invites you to shift into a broader mindset, one that allows for nuance, flexibility and deeper connection.

For instance, one of the questions below asks, "Do I want to build walls, or do I want to create connection?" On the surface, this might sound like wall-building is always a sign of being stuck. But in certain contexts, like recovering from abuse or ending a harmful relationship, building walls can be a vital, Self-led act of protection. In those moments, creating distance isn't about adversarial thinking; it's about reclaiming safety. These prompts aren't about denying the value of boundaries or certainty; they are helping you discern whether a mindset is narrowing your options or expanding your Self-leadership.

The next time you feel stuck in one of the Shame Triangle mindsets, take a breath and consider the following shifts:

From an Adversarial Mindset to a Restorative Mindset

- Am I here to win or to understand?
- Am I judging or getting curious?
- Am I blaming or owning my part?
- Am I building walls or creating connection?
- Am I seeking punishment or inviting repair?

From Binary Thinking to a Non-Dual Mindset

- Am I stuck in either/or, or can I hold both/and?
- Can two truths exist side by side?
- Am I chasing certainty or making space for complexity?
- Am I feeling separate or also connected?
- Am I collapsing into one story or holding the full picture?

From a Fixed Mindset to a Growth Mindset

- Is this the end of the road or part of my becoming?
- Is this failure or feedback?
- Am I avoiding this or growing through it?
- Am I focused on limits or what's possible?
- Am I trying to be perfect or being real?

From an Expert Mindset to a Beginner's Mindset

- Am I proving or learning?
- Am I defending or discovering?
- Am I controlling or staying curious?
- Am I holding the answer or making room for insight?
- What shifts if I treat this like the first time?

The R's of Releasing Beliefs and Resonating with New Ones

In addition to these mindset pivots, we also want to offer several exercises for working with the difficult beliefs held by your Shame Triangle parts. Even as you begin to adopt a more open perspective, some parts of you may still feel weighed down by deeply held beliefs. The following exercises draw from the IFS concept of unburdening, as well as shamanic and nature-based practices. Each follows a core process of releasing limiting beliefs, guided by variations of the R's: Reconnect, Reveal, Remove, Release and Reclaim. The steps involve connecting with Self, identifying the beliefs you want to shed, releasing them through a transformative or symbolic act, and finally reclaiming the qualities and truths you want to embody. While the wording may differ, the goal remains the same: to free you from outdated, problem-saturated narratives and create space for more supportive truths.

We encourage you to try each exercise at least once to see which resonates most. After exploring them, continue with the method—or combination of methods—that feels most effective for you. Beliefs have a way of entrancing the mind and pulling other parts into their logic, making them feel inescapable. That's why staying connected to Self throughout this process is essential.

A Ball of Beliefs

Reconnect

Start by tuning in and centering in Self. If needed, unblend from any parts, asking them to externalize for this exercise. Invite the part you want to work with to come forward, meeting it with curiosity and openness.

Reveal

Ask the part what beliefs it is carrying. Pinpoint the specific negative beliefs the part is holding. Gently inquire:

- How did you come to hold these beliefs?
- Where did they originate?
- Who or what influenced you to believe this?
- What impact have these beliefs had on my life?

Listen with empathy. Validate how painful it must have been for this part to carry these beliefs for so long. Acknowledge that these beliefs were learned, not inherent, and that they can be released.

Remove

Imagine pulling out all the beliefs this part carries and forming them into a ball. The part may hold the ball in its hands, or it might let the ball float in front of it. The ball could be made of smoke, tar, light or any other substance. Take your time until all the beliefs are gathered into this ball.

Release

Have this part choose an element to release the ball to—earth to decompose, wind to dissolve, fire to transform or water to cleanse. As the ball is released, affirm its departure by saying, "I release this ball of beliefs to the [element]. I no longer carry them."

Pause for a few breaths. Feel the inner spaciousness without these beliefs. Notice the lightness in your body and the freedom in this part now that it has let go of these beliefs.

Reclaim

Identify the supportive beliefs and qualities that were overshadowed by the old ones. Mentally or verbally invite these qualities into you. Visualize them as seeds being planted within, knowing they will continue to grow in your life. Let these beliefs and qualities sink deep, resonating through your entire being. Imagine them expanding outward, influencing how you see yourself and how you move through the world.

Affirm this reclamation by saying: "I reclaim my [quality], and I welcome it fully into my life."

Close the Practice

Take a moment to breathe and integrate this shift. Thank the part for its willingness to release what no longer serves and embrace new possibilities. When you feel ready, gently bring your awareness back to the present moment.

Waterfall of New Beliefs

Reconnect

Start by centering yourself in Self. If needed, unblend from any parts by asking them to externalize for this exercise. Invite the part you want to work with to come forward, meeting it with curiosity and openness.

Reveal

Ask the part what beliefs it is carrying. Pinpoint the specific negative beliefs it holds. Gently inquire:
- How did you come to hold these beliefs?
- Where did they originate?
- Who or what influenced you to believe this?
- What impact have these beliefs had on my life?

Listen with compassion. Acknowledge how difficult it has been for this part to carry these beliefs. Recognize that they were learned, not inherent, and that they can be released.

Remove and Release

Visualize a radiant waterfall of pure, healing light in front of you. This light can be any color that feels cleansing and comforting. Step under the waterfall and feel the warm, soothing light cascading over you from head to toe.

As the light flows over you, imagine it dissolving and washing away the limiting beliefs this part has carried. See these beliefs lifting from your body, dissolving into the light and being carried away. With each breath, release anything that no longer serves you, allowing the waterfall to cleanse and transform these beliefs.

Affirm this release by saying: "I let go of these beliefs. They do not define me, and I no longer carry them."

Resonate

Now, shift your focus to what you want to embody. Identify the beliefs and qualities you are ready to embrace—self-love, confidence, peace, trust or anything else that resonates. Imagine the waterfall now flowing with these new beliefs, pouring into you. Feel the light infusing every part of your being with these qualities. Let them settle into you, vibrating at your core, aligning with your true Self. Picture them expanding outward, influencing how you see yourself and how you move through the world.

Affirm this shift by saying: "I welcome these new beliefs into my life. I embody them fully."

Close the Practice

Take a few breaths and allow this transformation to settle in. When you feel ready, gently return to the present, carrying these new beliefs forward with you.

Root Down and Receive Up

Reconnect

Begin by centering yourself in Self. If needed, unblend from any parts, asking them to externalize for this exercise. Invite the part you want to work with to come forward, meeting it with curiosity and openness.

Root Down

Visualize roots extending from the base of this part and reaching deep into the earth. Feel these roots anchoring you, providing stability and support. Imagine them spreading wide and deep, connecting to the earth's nurturing and transformative energy. As these roots expand, feel the earth's grounding presence rising up through them, offering a sense of calm, strength and belonging.

Reveal

Ask the part what beliefs it carries and wants to release. Listen with compassion. Acknowledge how difficult it has been for this part to carry these beliefs for so long. Ask:
- Where did these beliefs come from?
- How did you learn them?
- What impact have they had on my life?

Recognize that these beliefs were learned, not inherent, and that they can be released.

Release to the Earth

Visualize these old beliefs flowing down through the roots into the earth. See the earth receiving them, breaking them down and transforming them. Just as nature composts and renews, the earth absorbs these beliefs and recycles their energy. Feel their weight lifting from you, leaving space for something new.

Affirm this release by saying: "I let these beliefs go. The earth receives them, transforms them, and I am free."

Receive Up

Now, imagine the earth sending up renewed energy, filled with supportive beliefs and qualities. They flow upward through the roots, filling you with strength, clarity and confidence. Feel this new energy rising into you, replenishing and healing. Let it spread through your entire being, solidifying your connection to Self. Notice the shift—the openness, the lightness, the possibility of seeing yourself in a new way.

Affirm this shift by saying: "I welcome these new beliefs. I am grounded, strong and open to growth."

Close the Practice

Take a few deep breaths and allow this transformation to settle in. Feel the support of the earth beneath you and the openness within you. When you feel ready, gently return to the present, carrying this renewed energy with you.

Tuning In to Preferred Beliefs

Like a tuning fork, we can attune ourselves to the beliefs we want to embody, allowing them to vibrate within us and expand outward.

Reconnect

Begin by centering yourself in Self. Take a few deep breaths, letting any distractions or tensions settle. If needed, unblend from any parts and invite them to step back.

Resonate (or "Retune")

Imagine a tuning fork in the center of your body, representing the new beliefs you wish to embody—confidence, trust, self-love, peace or any other qualities that resonate with you. Visualize the fork being struck, sending out pure, clear vibrations through your entire being. Feel this frequency aligning every part of you with these beliefs. Let the vibrations ripple outward, dissolving any resistance and bringing your whole system into harmony with these truths.

Affirm this resonance by saying: "I am in tune with [belief], and I allow it to vibrate through me."

Radiate

As the vibration strengthens, feel it expanding beyond you. Picture waves of this energy flowing outward, influencing your thoughts, actions and presence in the world. Imagine these beliefs becoming a natural part of how you carry yourself, interact with others and move through life.

Affirm this expansion by saying: "This belief radiates from within me, shaping how I see myself and the world."

Close the Practice

Take a few breaths, feeling the stability of this resonance. When you feel ready, gently return to the present, carrying this attuned energy forward with you.

Δ

The mind is powerful—but it is not always right. It is not neutral. It is shaped by everything we have learned, everything we have been told, everything we have feared. If left to itself, the mind will repeat what is familiar, rather than what is true.

In this chapter, we explored how the Shame Triangle warps the mind, trapping us in limiting beliefs, harsh narratives and rigid ways of thinking. We have begun the work of shifting from adversarial, binary, expert and fixed thinking toward more expansive, Self-led perspectives. A Self-centered mind is not one that never rushes to conclusions, misinterprets, spins out in worst-case scenarios or clings to rigid beliefs. But when these mental habits inevitably show up, the Self-centered mind knows how to pause, question and make space for new perspectives.

Now that we've explored how the Shame Triangle operates through the body, heart and mind—and how each center can be brought back into alignment through Self-leadership—we shift to a new layer of this work. What happens when the Shame Triangle doesn't originate within us, but is inherited from those around us? And how do we bring everything we've explored so far into a cohesive, Self-led system where these parts can relate to one another in a new way? The next chapters begin to answer these questions.

CHAPTER 10
WHEN YOUR SHAME TRIANGLE ISN'T YOURS

Our Shame Triangle is never entirely our own. Throughout this book, we have emphasized how the Shame Triangle is *internalized* from the world around us. Now, we explore when it is *inherited*. From family dynamics to historical traumas, beliefs and fears can be passed down across generations, shaping our inner landscape in ways we don't always recognize. These inherited burdens can feel like they belong to us, even when they originate from experiences we have not personally endured.

A fear of scarcity that lingers long after financial stability is reached. A sense of unworthiness that seems disproportionate to personal experience. Cycles of anxiety, addiction or self-doubt that mirror those of people who came before us. These patterns aren't always personal struggles—they can also be imprints of past pain carried forward in families and communities.

There are many ways to describe inherited trauma, and different fields use different terms to explain it:
- **Ancestral trauma:** Trauma from past generations that continues to affect descendants, often linked to events like war, famine or displacement (Bowen 1978).

- **Intergenerational, multigenerational or transgenerational trauma:** Psychological wounds passed down through family lines, shaping coping mechanisms, stress responses and emotional patterns (Yehuda and Lehrner 2018). This trauma can include cycles of abuse, addiction or poverty-related stress.
- **Historical trauma:** Collective trauma experienced by a cultural or racial group, such as colonization, slavery or forced displacement, with lasting generational effects (Brave Heart 2000).
- **Inherited family trauma:** Personal and emotional burdens passed down from parents or grandparents, sometimes without direct awareness (Wolynn 2016).
- **Legacy burdens:** Unresolved traumas or limiting beliefs inherited from previous generations that shape how we see ourselves and the world (Schwartz and Sweezy 2020).
- **Collective trauma:** Widespread suffering from disasters, wars or societal oppression that influences group identity and emotional resilience (Hirschberger 2018).
- **Epigenetic inheritance:** A biological lens on inherited trauma that examines how life experiences, particularly stress and trauma, can alter gene expression across generations (Yehuda et al. 2016; Yehuda and Lehrner 2018). For example, research has shown that children of famine or Holocaust survivors often display distinct stress-hormone levels and epigenetic markers, suggesting that trauma in one generation can have measurable biological effects on the next.
- **Past life trauma:** A spiritual perspective that suggests experiences from previous lifetimes may shape current fears, patterns or emotional struggles (Weiss 1988). While this concept lies outside mainstream science, it is accepted in certain religious and spiritual traditions and explored in some forms of hypnotherapy.

All of these perspectives underscore that our Shame Triangle can be shaped by forces beyond our own direct experiences. Some of these forces are echoes of what came before, woven into our emotional and psychological makeup through family and cultural history. Events like persecution or tragedy can forge Shame Triangle parts whose origins we only partly understand. When these inherited beliefs and emotions remain unprocessed, they can influence our bodies, hearts and minds in both overt and subtle ways.

Some signs that you may be carrying a legacy burden are:
- You've done extensive self-healing, therapy or medical treatment, but certain emotional or physical symptoms persist.
- You struggle with deep shame, fear, anxiety or perfectionism that feels out of proportion to your personal experiences.
- You notice repeating patterns of addiction, relationship struggles or self-sabotage that mirror those of family members who came before you.
- A pattern of specific tragedies, losses or even ways of dying repeats in your family over generations.
- You have memories, emotions or dreams that feel connected to your ancestors or cultural lineage rather than your own lived experience.
- Your family history includes intergenerational trauma, secrecy or a lack of open conversation about the past.
- You identify as being energetically sensitive, psychic or an empath, which can make you more susceptible to carrying energies or burdens that are from someone else.
- You feel disconnected from your ancestry or cultural roots, as if a part of your identity is missing or blocked.
- You experience unexplained fears, phobias or aversions that don't seem connected to anything in your own life.

> **Jessica here!**

When I began exploring my own Inner Critics, I identified two distinct inner voices. The first adopted the stern, authoritative tone of a strict British boarding school teacher, preoccupied with propriety and respectability. This voice scrutinized my sexuality, body image and romantic relationships through a puritanical lens. It imposed rigid standards of decorum and restraint while shaming any expression that deviated from its narrow framework of what a "proper girl" should do or look like. The second voice carried a distinctly masculine energy, berating me around success, ambition and achievement. This voice embodied the stereotypical tough-guy persona often seen in mafia movies, complete with a thick Brooklyn accent. It zeroed in on my perceived failings with intense judgment, hurling comments like, "Who do you think you are? Get it together! What's the matter wit' you? You some kinda idiot or something?!"

Because I grew up in Brooklyn, it made sense that I had internalized this tough Brooklyn persona. But the British boarding school teacher was a figure from an environment I had never directly experienced—probably something I picked up from movies. Yet both voices, as dramatically different as they were, felt entirely real in my inner world, serving as internalized echoes of the judgments and expectations I had absorbed throughout my upbringing and socialization.

I also encountered a third Inner Critic voice that sounded just like my grandmother—the cadence, the tone, even the phrasing matched how she used to speak to me, and how I'd hear her talk to others when I was growing up. I tried everything I knew to work with this part, using all the methods in this book as well as EMDR therapy, but no matter what I did, this grandma-like Inner Critic wouldn't budge. It was as if I'd reached the edge of what these tools could do. Frustrated by my inability to change it, I had a realization: Maybe this voice wasn't merely my own

Inner Critic mimicking my grandmother, but something of hers that I had inadvertently inherited.

Having exhausted my usual approaches, I decided to shift to energetic exercises instead and decided to engage in a cord-cutting exercise (more on this exercise later in this chapter). I visualized my grandmother standing ten or fifteen feet away from me and asked the energetic cords between us to be revealed. There were many. Some looked like beams of light, others like octopus tentacles or fleshy appendages connecting us. The widest and most prominent cord between us was from her hip to mine. In my real life, I had a persistent pain in that hip—clicking and popping, too much tightness in some areas and too much laxity in others. I had done plenty of physical therapy and corrective exercise, but the relief was always temporary.

As I focused on that particular cord, I asked myself what was being held there. The intuitive answer I received was grief—hers, not mine. I knew she had had many losses she never fully dealt with, including the death of her five-year-old child and, a few years later, her husband. So this connection initially made sense to me. It felt like something unspoken had been passed down from her and stored in my body, waiting to be acknowledged. I asked for divine light to come down and perform a "spiritual surgery" to sever the cords that bound us. Some dissolved. Others were removed from us but still remained intact, so I sent them up to the sun to be transformed into useful energy. Then I asked for anything I was holding, known or unknown, that belonged to my grandmother, to be sent back to her. I visualized her grief leaving my hip and returning to her. Next, I requested that any parts of myself that were being held by her be returned to me. As this energetic exchange happened, we both lit up with the Self-energy that the other had been carrying. I thanked my grandmother, bowed to her and closed the exercise. After the exercise was complete, I was clear that I had been carrying

> her grief, but I wasn't yet sure how it connected to the Inner Critic I had experienced.
>
> The next time I saw my grandma, who was then in her 80s, I asked about her experience losing a child in her 30s. It was the first time she told me about the moment she learned of her child's death, and her description aligned precisely with what I had seen during the cord-cutting exercise. My grandma also shared additional details I hadn't known. After her daughter's death, her closest family members advised her to clean out the girl's room and move on. She didn't know how to grieve, and she didn't seem to be allowed to grieve either, so she imagined putting all of her feelings and pain into her pocket—right where my hip pain was—and never looking back. She also shared that in many ways it was easier to be angry than to allow the feelings of loss.
>
> In place of her grief, an angry critic arose to keep her from the vulnerability of feeling her unprocessed pain. Even though she could be incredibly sweet, she also had a fierce Outer Critic—a version of an Escaper that protected her from emotions she didn't feel safe to express. Unknowingly and unintentionally, she passed down both her unresolved pain and her critical voice to subsequent generations. Her grief, which had no space to be felt, had lodged itself in my body as physical pain, and her Critic, which kept her from breaking down, had become mine, too.

Both of us, Dave and Jessica, have encountered similar patterns in the people we work with. Some report that their Inner Critic sounds exactly like the voice of an abuser, while others recognize that their Shame and Escaper parts resemble specific figures from their past. Many people intuitively know that certain struggles they face actually belong to someone else. When doing parts work and asking a part how long it has been with them, it's not uncommon for the part to say it has always been there, originating at birth or even before—suggesting that it is inherited, rather than internalized. Additionally, many people have noticed that the intensity of their fears or emotional reactivity feels disproportionate to their actual lived experiences. One possibility is that these responses stem from intergenerational traumas and burdens. This response is particularly prevalent among those with a family history of war, genocide, enslavement or ethnic cleansing, even when these events occurred generations ago.

Furthermore, we've worked with people from historically marginalized communities who, despite not having experienced direct physical harm in this lifetime, still carry it in their bodies as if they had. Some people even recount memories of past lives where they have been tortured, exiled or killed for their beliefs or identities, while others have traumatic memories of being on other planets or in different dimensions that impact their lives today. The definitive truth of any of these claims is not important here. In our experience with different ancestral healing modalities, the important thing is to honor what may have been inherited (instead of judging it to be fabricated) and offer a means through which someone can heal and release any legacy burdens they are holding. Inherited traumas can leave imprints on our minds, bodies and energetic fields, shaping our present-day realities, even when the origins of these traumas cannot be empirically proven.

Many different ancient traditions and contemporary healing modalities recognize that we are not isolated individuals, but part of a vast web of interconnected relationships that span time and space. Fortunately, healing is possible, and by addressing ancestral wounds, we not only heal ourselves but also our lineage—both past and future. We can break cycles of suffering and pave the way for future generations to thrive. Several modalities offer pathways to this kind of healing, each providing unique approaches to addressing and releasing these heavy burdens.

Here are some approaches used to address inherited burdens and ancestral trauma:
- **Family constellations work (Bert Hellinger):** This experiential, group-based practice helps individuals uncover hidden family dynamics and inherited traumas.

Participants represent different family members or relational dynamics, physically mapping out a client's family system. Through dialogue and movement, unconscious entanglements and multigenerational patterns come to light, offering insight and resolution for long-standing struggles.
- **Legacy unburdening:** A specialized IFS technique that explores inherited burdens within a specific lineage. Through guided dialogue and visualization, you invite the ancestor who originally carried the burden—whether a known relative or someone from generations past—to step forward. By acknowledging what was passed down and working with this ancestor to release it, you also reclaim strengths and positive qualities that may have been overshadowed by these inherited patterns.
- **Shamanic ancestral healing:** These practices involve connecting with ancestral guides and using rituals, ceremonies, soul retrieval or ancestral altars to engage with and release inherited burdens. Through shamanic journeying or direct communication with ancestral spirits, individuals seek guidance and healing across non-ordinary realms.
- **Somatic experiencing (Peter Levine):** A body-focused approach that helps release trauma stored in the nervous system, including inherited trauma patterns. Somatic experiencing uses mindfulness, breathwork and gentle movements to renegotiate traumatic activation, helping to restore a sense of safety and self-regulation in the body.
- **Systemic constellations work:** Similar to family constellations work, this group-based practice maps out relationships within a family or ancestral system. Representatives stand in for family members or aspects of a client's lineage, revealing hidden influences that shape present-day struggles. Through interaction and repositioning, the system is rebalanced, shifting patterns rooted in the family's history.

- **Generational healing (Mark Wolynn):** This approach focuses on identifying unconscious family imprints and transforming patterns passed down through generations. Techniques may include dialogue with earlier ancestors, guided visualization and somatic practices to address inherited trauma at its roots.
- **Epigenetic healing:** Based on research into how trauma can alter gene expression across generations, this approach works to rewire inherited biological patterns. Modalities such as energy psychology use tapping, breathwork and focused intention to shift deep-seated stress responses linked to ancestral trauma (Yehuda et al. 2016; Yehuda and Lehrner 2018).
- **Ritual and ceremony:** Many cultural and spiritual traditions offer structured ways to honor ancestors and release inherited burdens. These may include prayer, spiritual or physical cleansing, offerings or seasonal observances that mark transitions in the natural world. Rituals may also center around birth, death and grieving—times when the veil between generations feels especially thin. Engaging in ceremony can help acknowledge what has been carried, invite guidance from those who came before, and create space for release, connection and healing.

Exercises

The following exercises help us recognize what was never truly ours to carry, release ancestral wounds, and reclaim the strengths and wisdom that may have been overshadowed. Healing legacy burdens can happen in a moment or unfold slowly over time. There's no right pace, so allow space for whatever arises. If you start to feel overwhelmed, pause and return when you're ready. If strong emotions or memories surface, stay present by focusing on your breath and tuning into the sensations in your body—this can help ground you and prevent emotional flooding.

After each exercise, consider journaling, sketching or recording a voice memo. Capturing your experience in some way can help you process and integrate new insights. If these practices bring up particularly intense feelings, seeking professional support may be helpful. A therapist or practitioner who specializes in ancestral healing or trauma work can provide guidance and create a safe space for deeper exploration.

Reclaiming Your Energetic Sovereignty (Cord Cutting)

This exercise is designed to help you detach from and release any Shame Triangle parts or other inherited burdens you've taken on from someone else in your life. Whether it's a critical voice, ancestral trauma or a negative pattern that doesn't feel like it's truly yours, the goal is to reclaim your energetic sovereignty and realign with your authentic Self.

Ground Yourself and Connect with Self

Sit comfortably in a quiet space where you won't be disturbed. Take a few deep breaths to center yourself, feeling your body supported by the surface beneath you. Allow any parts that aren't directly involved in this exercise to step back or unblend. Connect with Self.

Visualize the Influential Person

Bring to mind the individual, group or ancestor from whom you sense you've inherited a burden or internalized a negative voice. If your focus is specifically on an internalized critic, you might picture the person whose criticisms shaped that part of you. Imagine this person's energetic presence standing before you, separate from your own body. Simply notice the sensations and emotions that arise without judging or rushing to alter them.

Reveal the Energetic Ties

Ask to see any energetic cords, ties or connections linking you to this person or pattern. Invite insight about how and why these cords formed. Were they created through repeated criticisms, ancestral trauma or a sense of responsibility for someone else's pain?

Cut the Cords

Use your breath to guide the cutting process. With each exhale, focus on detaching or dissolving any cords you discover. You can use some of these options to assist the cord cutting.
- **Laser beam:** Visualize a concentrated beam of light slicing cleanly through the cords, removing them from both your body and the other person's.
- **Dissolving solution:** Imagine a gentle liquid washing over the cords, causing them to dissolve until no trace remains.
- **Spiritual assistance:** Call upon any supportive beings or guides to remove the cords with care and precision.

Release the Cords

Once the cords are detached, choose how to send them back to the elements to complete their transformation. This act symbolizes the full release and neutralization of their influence over you.
- **Bury in earth:** Visualize burying the cords in the soil and allowing the earth to compost and transform this energy into nutrients that nourish new growth.
- **Send to the sun:** Imagine sending these cords up to the sun, where they are incinerated and converted into radiant energy that diffuses harmlessly into the vastness of space.
- **Release into the ocean:** Picture these cords being washed away into the ocean, where the salt water cleanses and disperses their energy and allows it to flow away with the tides.

- **Release into the wind:** Visualize letting go of the cords into the wind, where they unravel and are carried far away, dispersing into air and sky until they lose all form and dissolve.
- **Offer to fire:** Imagine placing the cords into a fire, where they are consumed and transformed by the flames.

Continue focusing on release until you feel this step is complete.

Exchange Energy

State that you are returning any energy or life force belonging to other people that you have been holding, intentionally or unintentionally. Imagine this energy is leaving your body and gravitating back to the other person for them to receive. If you'd like, you can state, either silently or aloud, "All that is yours that I have been carrying, I return to you" or "This is no longer mine to hold, and I return it to you."

Then ask that any of your Self-energy or life force that the other has been holding be returned to you. Imagine this energy leaving their body, gravitating back to you and reabsorbing into your body. If you'd like, you can state, either silently or aloud, "All that is mine, please return to me. I reclaim my sovereignty, my truth."

Affirm and Close the Practice

Take some deep breaths and affirm: "I am realigned with my own vibration. Only my inner wisdom guides me from now on." Close the exercise by thanking the other person for the lessons they provided and wishing them well on their journey.

IFS-Inspired Legacy Unburdening Exercise

This exercise draws on the legacy unburdening approach within IFS, as developed by Anne Sinko (2017). In her method, the facilitator guides a person to identify the ancestor who first carried the burden and then moves through each generation in the lineage. While this process is typically done with a trained practitioner to allow for deeper facilitation and safety, the version presented here is adapted for self-guided work. Rather than relying on an external facilitator and relating to each person in your lineage, you will treat the inherited burden like a "part" within you, dialoguing with it directly. This approach retains the transformative essence of legacy unburdening—uncovering ancestral wounds, reclaiming positive qualities and restoring wholeness—while offering a structured way to practice on your own.

Ground and Connect with Your Self

Begin by taking several deep, calming breaths. Allow your body to settle into a comfortable position, and bring your awareness fully into the present moment. Settle into Self-energy. If needed, unblend from any parts that are not involved in this exercise.

Identify the Legacy Burden

Bring to mind a specific issue, pattern or challenge that you suspect is rooted in your family or ancestral legacies. Notice any thoughts, emotions, body sensations or imagery that arise as you focus on it.

Personify the Legacy Burden

Sense if there is a legacy burden part carrying this inherited imprint or wound. Imagine it externalizing. Let it stand before you, so you can engage with it more directly.

Connect with the Burden Part

With curiosity and compassion, inform this part that you wish to understand it. Reassure it that your intention is to heal together. Invite the part to share whatever it wants you to know about the burden it carries.
- How did you come to carry this legacy burden?
- What memories, emotions or beliefs do you hold?

- What were you trying to accomplish—even in extreme or maladaptive ways?
- How have you attempted to help or protect me?

Transform the Burden with the Elements

Invite the legacy burden part to pull out the burden (which may appear as a dark mass, heavy object or any symbolic form). Ask the part which element—fire, earth, air or water—can best transform it. Visualize the part handing the burden over to that element, allowing it to be burned, composted, dispersed or washed away. Take a moment to sense any shift as the burden dissipates.

Recognize Positive Qualities

Encourage the part to identify and honor qualities that were overshadowed by this inherited wound—perhaps resilience, wisdom or love. Allow it to fully absorb these qualities. If it feels right, you too can welcome them into your body, heart and mind, envisioning this newly freed energy lighting up within you.

Reintegrate the Part

Now that the burden has been released, invite the part to take on a new, supportive role aligned with your Self-energy. Acknowledge its past efforts to protect or help, and affirm that you value its gifts. See or sense it reintegrating within you, carrying the positive qualities it has just reclaimed.

Close the Exercise

Breathe deeply, noticing what may have shifted inside. Offer gratitude to all parts of you for carrying these burdens, and honor the healing that has occurred. When you feel complete, gently open your eyes or bring your attention back to your surroundings. You may wish to journal or reflect on this experience, noting any insights or feelings of release and renewal.

Collective Ancestral Unburdening

In some legacy unburdening sessions, a particular wound or belief doesn't belong exclusively to one branch of the family tree. You may discover that both sides of your lineage—parents, grandparents, aunts, uncles and even more distant ancestors—share the same or similar burden. In these cases, rather than working with only one line, you can invite all ancestors connected to this issue to come forward collectively. By gathering and transforming the burden as a group, each generation participates in releasing what they've been carrying and welcomes in the positive qualities that have been overshadowed. Below is a step-by-step guide to help you facilitate a collective generational unburdening.

Connect with Self

Find a quiet, comfortable space and take a few grounding breaths. Connect with your Self-energy. Invite any parts not involved in this particular exercise to step back momentarily.

Set a Clear Intention

You are here to work with an inherited pattern or belief that spans multiple lines of your family or ancestral system.

Identify the Shared Family Burden

Bring to mind a specific issue, pattern or belief that feels ingrained and likely shared by multiple relatives (e.g., chronic anxiety, scarcity mindset, addiction, etc).

Tune In

Connect with the sensations, emotions or images that arise. Ask internally: How many sides of my family might hold this burden? Does this come from one or both sides of my lineage?

Silently inquire: How far back does this burden extend? Notice any impressions, images or intuitive senses of earlier generations. You might sense it goes back to grandparents, great-grandparents or even further.

Invite All Affected Ancestors

Imagine you're standing in a wide, open space. Call forth all the ancestors who contributed to or were affected by this same burden. Visualize them arriving in groups—siblings, cousins, spouses and extended family—and gathering themselves in generations. Trust whatever imagery or sense of presence emerges. If it feels right, welcome anyone impacted by this pattern, not only blood relatives but also close partners or in-laws who might have carried it.

Gather and Acknowledge the Burden

Ask the members of your generation to gather whatever aspects of the burden they've been holding into a central mass or ball. This could appear as darkness, weight, smoke or any other symbolic representation. Encourage them to share, in whatever form they can, how this burden has affected their lives. Allow time for each member to place their portion of the burden into this collective mass.

Move Through the Generations

Once the first generation has contributed their portion of the burden, invite the next (parents, aunts, uncles, etc.) to step forward. Repeat the same process: They acknowledge and place their share of the burden into the growing mass. Continue until you've reached the most distant generation you sense is involved, whether grandparents, great-grandparents or further back.

Transform the Burden

Ask the final generation (or the entire gathering collectively) which element—fire, earth, air or water—can best transform this burden. Visualize them offering the mass to that element.

- **Fire** may burn it away into smoke and ash, freeing its energy.
- **Earth** can absorb and compost it into fertile soil.
- **Air** might carry it off in a powerful wind, dispersing it.
- **Water** can dissolve and purify it, washing it away.

Reflect on the Positive Qualities

As the burden is released and transformed, encourage each generation to recognize the strengths, gifts and wisdom they can now embody without the burden overshadowing them. Encourage them to fully receive and embody these positive legacies—qualities like resilience, creativity, love, courage or anything else that naturally belongs to them. Imagine these qualities filling and illuminating each person, lighting them up from within.

Receive the Gifts

When the time feels right, see these ancestors offering their gifts to you—passing them forward with love. Allow yourself to receive them fully, welcoming the support of your lineage in its healed form.

Reintegrate

Thank each generation of ancestors for their willingness to unburden and heal. Sense or watch as they collectively integrate these renewed qualities. If you like, you can envision them returning to their places in your ancestral line, now freer and more at peace.

Close the Exercise

Take a moment to notice how you feel. Allow any parts within you to relax and absorb the shift that has occurred. You might say a short statement of gratitude or prayer, honoring the transformation that took place. Gently come back to the present, taking a few deep breaths. If it feels right, journal or record your impressions of the process.

Solo Family Constellation Exercise

This guided exercise adapts the principles of family constellation work, which is traditionally conducted in a group setting using live representatives, to an individual practice. Here, you'll use objects or figures to represent family members and potential legacy burdens. By visually arranging and interacting with these placeholders, you can gain insight into the intergenerational dynamics that shape your life and begin to untangle inherited patterns that no longer serve you.

You will need several small objects or figures (stones, dolls, chess pieces, paper cutouts, etc.) to represent family members and significant relationships.

Set Up Your Space

Choose a quiet area where you can lay out your constellation without interruptions. Gather your objects and assign each one to represent a specific family member, including yourself.

Set an Intention

Before placing your objects, set an intention for the exercise. Your focus might be understanding a family dynamic, gaining clarity on a personal struggle or uncovering hidden influences in your lineage.

Put Yourself in the Center

Place the figure that represents you in the center of your space. Intuitively place the other figures around you based on their relationship to you and each other. Don't overthink their placement—trust your instincts.

Observe the Dynamics

Step back and notice how the figures are arranged. Observe distances—who is close to you, and who is farther away? Notice the directions they are facing—are they looking toward or away from you or each other?

Identify a Figure that Carries a Family Burden

The burden might represent sadness, conflict, guilt or unresolved trauma. Choose an additional object to symbolize this burden and place it near the figure carrying it to represent externalizing the burden.

Ask What They Feel

Silently or aloud, ask the figures what they feel, why they carry these burdens and what they need to release them. If it feels right, adjust the placement of the figures—turning them to face each other, bringing them closer together or farther apart, or even introducing new objects to represent support or transformation. Allow the constellation to shift in a way that feels more aligned, balanced or revealing.

Reflect and Close the Exercise

Once you feel the constellation has reached a meaningful state, step back and reflect. Journal about your observations, emotions and insights. Note any shifts in your understanding or feelings about your family dynamics. Thank the figures for their role in your exploration. Consciously gather the objects, acknowledging the work that has been done.

Somatic Exercise for Releasing Inherited Trauma

This exercise helps you connect with and release inherited trauma stored in the body. By tuning into sensations, calling on ancestral support and allowing movement and breath to facilitate release, you can begin to shift patterns passed down through your lineage. Move through the steps at your own pace.

Ground and Connect with Self

Find a comfortable place to sit or lie down. Close your eyes and take a few deep breaths. Connect with Self-energy. Feel the support of the ground beneath you. Notice where your body makes contact with the surface beneath you and allow yourself to settle into the present moment.

Set an intention for this session, such as healing inherited trauma, releasing stored tension from your lineage or bringing more ease into your body.

Do a Body Scan and Notice Sensory Awareness

Slowly bring your attention to different parts of your body, starting at your feet and moving up to your head. Notice any areas of tension, discomfort or numbness.

Pay close attention to any sensations that feel *different*—heaviness, tightness, pressure, warmth, coolness or a sense of constriction. If emotions surface, simply acknowledge them without judgment.

If a particular area feels tense, place a hand over it and breathe into it. Allow the sensation to be there without forcing it to change.

Identify the Inherited Energy

As you tune in, ask yourself: Does this sensation feel like mine, or does it seem older than me? You can also ask your body to show you where it is holding inherited burdens.

If an image, memory or emotion arises, trust what comes up. You may recall a family story, a specific ancestor or an event you weren't present for but somehow feel connected to.

Imagine gathering this inherited energy into a symbolic shape, color or object within your body. There's no right or wrong—just notice what form it takes.

Call in Ancestral Support

Now, invite in the benevolent ancestors—the ones who carry wisdom, love and healing. These may be specific relatives you know, or simply those in your lineage who have your best interests at heart.

Picture them surrounding you, offering their presence, warmth and strength. Feel their support as they stand beside you, ready to help release what no longer serves you.

If it feels right, allow yourself to connect with them. You might sense a message, a feeling or simply their witnessing presence. Let them be here with you.

Release Through Breath, Movement and Expression

Picture a warm, gentle light surrounding the area where this energy is stored. As you breathe, let the light soften and loosen the sensation.

Begin to move your body intuitively—roll your shoulders, stretch your arms, shake out your hands or sway side to side. Let the movement flow naturally and be as big or small as you need.

If emotions or sounds arise, allow them to move through you. You may feel the need to sigh, hum, exhale deeply or let out a sound. If shaking or trembling occurs, trust it—it's your body's way of completing what was once frozen in time.

As you move, visualize the energy lifting and leaving your body, dissolving into the earth, wind, water or fire—whichever element feels right for transformation. Feel your ancestors witnessing and supporting you in this release. Know that you are not doing this alone.

Reclaim and Restore

As the release process completes, take a few moments to sit quietly. Notice any shifts.

Place a hand on the area of your body where the release occurred. Imagine this space now filling with your Self-energy, with pure, healing light flowing into it. The space where the inherited burden once was is now fully inhabited by your own energy. Feel the warmth, strength and clarity of your own essence settling in, restoring balance. Feel yourself connected, stable and fully present in your body.

Gratitude and Closing

Thank your ancestors for their support and presence. If there's anything you'd like to say to them, do so now. Express gratitude to your body for carrying you through this experience.

Meeting Your Benevolent Ancestors

This exercise guides you through a visualization practice to connect with your ancestors and receive their wisdom and guidance. It can be approached from a spiritual perspective or simply as a creative, imaginative process, whichever resonates with you.

Create a Personal Space

Find a quiet, undisturbed area where you feel comfortable. Enhance the space with items that have personal meaning—candles, photos, natural objects or anything that helps you feel connected.

Ground and Center Yourself

Take several deep, slow breaths to anchor yourself in the present moment. Allow your mind to settle and your body to relax. Connect into Self-energy.

Invite Support

Whether you choose a spiritual framework or a purely imaginative one, invite supportive energies into your space. You might call on spiritual guides, the divine or simply your inner wisdom. State your intention to connect with benevolent ancestral energies, ensuring you feel both safe and supported throughout the exercise.

Visualize Your Ancestors' Home

Close your eyes and visualize traveling to a realm where your ancestors reside. This realm might appear as an ancient forest, a luminous open space, a cave, a floating island or any landscape that feels right for you. Let your intuition guide the journey.

Be Open to Their Presence

When you arrive, be open to the presence of an ancestor. If you are greeted, you may ask, "Are you my ancestor?"

If you don't see or sense anything initially, ask for a supportive ancestor to come forward. This could be a known relative or an ancestral guide you've never met before. Trust whatever images, sensations or impressions arise as you welcome them into your awareness.

Initiate a Respectful Dialogue

Greet the presence with gratitude and respect, then share what's in your heart—whether it's questions, struggles or hopes. Listen to their response, allowing the conversation to flow naturally without judgment.

Receive Their Guidance

Your ancestor may offer insights, symbols or memories related to your situation. Stay receptive to whatever arises and note any teachings or impressions that feel significant.

Give Thanks

Express sincere thanks to the ancestral presence for their guidance. If it feels appropriate, offer a symbolic token of gratitude—such as a flower, a bow or a meaningful object—to honor the exchange.

Close the Connection

When you feel ready, begin to bring your awareness back to the present moment. Allow the imagery of the ancestral realm to fade gradually as you reconnect with your physical surroundings.

Δ

Not every aspect of our Shame Triangle stems from personal experience. Many of the patterns we carry have been passed down through generations—embedded in our family systems and cultural histories, often without our conscious awareness. These inherited burdens shape the way our internal parts function, reinforcing beliefs and reactions that may not have begun with us. By engaging in these practices, you have the opportunity to untangle these patterns for yourself and initiate a process of healing beyond yourself. As we transform our own Shame Triangle, we also shift what gets passed forward, creating the possibility for future generations to live with greater freedom. This work is central to the journey described in this book—to understand, embrace and ultimately move beyond the parts of ourselves shaped by external forces so that we can step fully into who we truly are.

CHAPTER 11
BRINGING OUR SHAME TRIANGLE PARTS TOGETHER INTO THE SELF-LOVE TRIANGLE

Thus far, we've worked with the Shame Triangle parts individually. Now, we arrive at an important juncture. Having unburdened their wounds and limiting beliefs, these parts are ready to engage with one another in entirely new ways—ways that transcend the old dynamics that once bound them. With Self in the lead, you can now facilitate a dialogue between these parts, helping them repair their relationships and integrate into a more cohesive, supportive system. This is a vital step, because healing our parts in isolation isn't sufficient—true transformation happens when we also repair the relationships between them and restore a sense of internal unity. When your parts move from opposition to collaboration, they shift from the Shame Triangle into the Self-Love Triangle, forming a more harmonious inner world.

Our approach to facilitating these conversations is inspired by the Restorative Relationship Conversation model developed by Dave to help people navigate interpersonal conflicts in a way that is relational rather than adversarial. His model is based on restorative justice principles, which offer an alternative to punitive, blame-driven approaches. Instead of focusing on retribution, restorative justice emphasizes repair, accountability and relational healing—a framework that prioritizes connection over punishment. At its core, restorative work is built on the understanding that humans are wired for relationship. Just as we need food, water and shelter to survive, we also need meaningful and secure relationships to thrive. When relationships are disrupted—whether with others or within ourselves—our well-being suffers.

Typically, restorative practices are used to repair harm between people. But here, we apply these same principles to the relationships between our internal parts. Just as external conflicts require a safe space for resolution, our internal dialogues must take place in an environment of safety, willingness and respect. In the RRC process, we create a structured and intentional space so that all perspectives can be heard, acknowledged and understood. Instead of blame and defensiveness, the focus is on personal responsibility—recognizing the impact of past behaviors while allowing room for transformation. In the context of parts work, this means supporting our parts to recognize their past roles and interactions, while also helping them move forward in a way that fosters cooperation and trust.

A core element of restorative dialogue is active listening, where each voice is given space to express itself without being dismissed or attacked. With internal parts work, this allows Shame, the Inner Critic and Escapers to communicate their experiences, express the pain they have carried and acknowledge how they have affected one another. Rather than forcing parts into agreement, the goal is to create a foundation for mutual understanding, allowing them to shift into more constructive relationships. The final stage of RRC is cocreating a new way forward. In external conflicts, this means agreeing on steps to repair harm and restore trust. Internally, this means guiding parts to establish new relational agreements—ones that allow them to function in healthier ways that serve the system as a whole. By integrating these restorative principles, we give our parts the opportunity to evolve beyond their outdated roles and become active participants in our healing.

In the exercises that follow, you'll facilitate a reconciliation between your parts, allowing them to interact in their updated forms. The process begins with one-on-one dialogues between parts, followed by a collective unburdening where all parts come together. Some shifts may happen quickly, while others will take more time. Just as two cats who have never met must first get acquainted from opposite sides of a door—sniffing, observing, getting used to each other before they can be in the same room—your parts may also need time to adjust. Simply bringing them together and allowing them to interact in a new way is an essential first step.

For example, the Inner Critic, now evolving into the Inner Coach, may recognize the harm it has caused Shame and genuinely express remorse. Shame, in turn, may be able to hear this apology and welcome the new dynamic with relief and openness. However, this isn't always the case. Shame may instead feel anger or distrust; it may need time to process the shift. In these moments, it's important to affirm that Shame has every right to feel this way and to take the time it needs. It may take more than one dialogue between them to rebuild trust and shift the dynamic.

Similarly, the Inner Critic may not yet feel comfortable trusting an Escaper's transformation into an Inner Nurturer. Depending on the type of Escaper it recalls dealing with, the Inner Critic may need real proof of change before it can let go of its old policing role. But as the Inner Critic transitions into the Inner Coach, it can begin to support the Inner Nurturer instead of controlling it—offering encouragement rather than judgment. These parts are not only learning to trust each other in new ways, but they also now have Self in leadership as a source of support that wasn't present before. Self ensures that no part has to carry the full weight of responsibility alone.

What matters most is that the parts begin to recognize that things are shifting. They don't need to become best friends overnight, but they do need to acknowledge that they no longer have to work against each other. Over time, these dialogues create the foundation for true internal collaboration, where each part can operate in a way that strengthens the whole.

Because these parts are still in transition, you'll see them referred to by both their old and emerging names, such as Inner Critic/Coach, Shame/Raw Experience or Escaper/Inner Nurturer. This reflects the reality that transformation is a process, not a flip of a switch. Naming the parts this way helps us honor both where they've been and what they're becoming, as they begin relating to one another in entirely new ways. Since there may be multiple Escaper parts that relate to the same Inner Critic part or Shame part, you can repeat these exercises for each Escaper to support their individual transformation and integration.

Repair Processes

Repair Process Between the Inner Critic/Coach and Shame/Raw Experience

Connect with Self-Energy: Begin by grounding yourself in Self-energy. Ensure that you are present, clear, calm, open, curious and ready to facilitate the dialogue. If any other parts jump in or need attention before beginning the conversation between the Inner Critic/Coach and Shame/Raw Experience, take a moment to tend to them and reassure them as needed.

Invite the Parts Forward: Call forward both the Inner Critic/Coach and Shame/Raw Experience. Let them know that you are here to support a repair conversation and help them build a better relationship. If needed, reassure Shame/Raw Experience that you are protecting it and that the old version of the Inner Critic is no longer in control.

Inner Critic/Coach Acknowledges Past Treatment: The Inner Critic/Coach speaks first, acknowledging how it has mistreated Shame in the past. From Self, encourage it to take responsibility for the ways it has been harmful and offer appreciation for its willingness to be accountable.

Shame/Raw Experience Shares Its Experience and Impact: Shame/Raw Experience then shares its experience—expressing what it felt like to be on the receiving end of the Inner Critic's actions and how those behaviors have affected it. From Self, offer appreciation or empathy for its willingness to be vulnerable.

Inner Critic/Coach Apologizes and Commits to Change: Now, invite the Inner Critic/Coach to respond to what it has just heard. It should acknowledge the specific impact that Shame/Raw Experience described, demonstrating that it has truly listened and understands the harm it caused. From this place, the Inner Critic/Coach offers a genuine apology and explains how it has changed and/or is changing. It can share its new role, its positive protective intentions, its commitment to a more constructive relationship and how it intends to function differently moving forward. (If the Inner Critic/Coach struggles with this step, you can pause and guide it through the process.)

Shame/Raw Experience Expresses Needs and Sets Boundaries: Shame/Raw Experience now has the opportunity to express any needs or set boundaries that will allow for a more supportive and respectful dynamic. If trust still needs to be built, ask both parts what they need from each other moving forward to help establish that trust.

Close the Process: Thank both parts for showing up in this process. Invite them to acknowledge each other in a closing gesture that feels right—this could be a verbal thank you, a handshake, a bow, a hug, a nod, etc. Offer any parting words that bring closure and reinforce the shift toward a more relational and cooperative connection.

Repair Process Between an Escaper/Inner Nurturer and Shame/Raw Experience

Connect with Self-Energy: Begin by grounding yourself in Self-energy, ensuring that you are present, clear, calm, open, curious and ready to facilitate the dialogue. If any other parts step in or need reassurance before starting the conversation between the Escaper/Inner Nurturer and Shame/Raw Experience, take a moment to tend to them.

Invite the Parts Forward: Call both the Escaper/Inner Nurturer and Shame/Raw Experience into the conversation. Let them know you are here to support a repair dialogue and foster a stronger, healthier relationship between them.

Escaper/Inner Nurturer Acknowledges Past Treatment: The Escaper/Inner Nurturer speaks first, acknowledging how it has treated Shame in the past. Encourage it to take responsibility, especially for the ways it has turned away rather than toward Shame/Raw Experience, and the unintended harm that it has caused. From Self, offer appreciation for its willingness to be accountable.

Shame/Raw Experience Shares Its Experience and Impact: Shame/Raw Experience now shares its experience—describing what it has felt like to be ignored, dismissed or abandoned by the Escaper and how that avoidance has affected it. From Self, offer appreciation or empathy for its willingness to express itself.

Escaper/Inner Nurturer Apologizes and Commits to Change: Invite the Escaper/Inner Nurturer to respond to what it has just heard, acknowledging the specific impact that Shame/Raw Experience described. This helps to demonstrate that it has truly listened and understands the harm caused. From this place, the Escaper/Inner Nurturer offers a genuine apology and explains how it has shifted its role. It can share its commitment to turning toward Shame/Raw Experience rather than avoiding it, offering nurturing and care instead of neglect, and how it intends to function moving forward. (If the Escaper/Inner Nurturer struggles with this step, you can pause and guide it through the process.)

Shame/Raw Experience Expresses Needs and Sets Boundaries: Shame/Raw Experience now has the opportunity to express any needs or set boundaries to ensure a more supportive and respectful relationship. If trust still needs to be built, ask both parts what they need from each other moving forward to strengthen that trust.

Close the Process: Thank both parts for showing up in this process. Invite them to acknowledge each other in a closing gesture that feels right—this could be a verbal thank you, a handshake, a bow, a hug, a nod, etc. Offer any parting words that bring closure and reinforce the shift toward a more relational and supportive connection.

Repair Process Between the Inner Critic/Coach and the Escaper/Inner Nurturer

Connect with Self-Energy: Begin by grounding yourself in Self-energy, ensuring that you are present, clear, calm, open, curious and ready to facilitate the dialogue. If any other parts step in or need reassurance before starting the conversation between the Inner Coach and the Inner Nurturer, take a moment to tend to them before proceeding.

Invite the Parts Forward: Call both the Inner Critic/Coach and Escaper/Inner Nurturer into the conversation. Let them know this is a safe and supportive space for a reparative and collaborative dialogue.

Acknowledge the Past Dynamic: The Inner Critic/Coach speaks first, acknowledging how it used criticism and judgment in an attempt to drive improvement or prevent failure. It reflects on how these strategies may have activated the Escaper's avoidance patterns, creating an unhelpful cycle. The Escaper/Inner Nurturer then acknowledges its role—recognizing that, in the past, it used avoidance as a coping strategy in response to the Inner Critic/Coach's pressure. It explains that its intention was to protect and soothe, even if it sometimes led to disengagement.

Both Parts Share Their Experience of the Other: Now, each part has the opportunity to share how they experienced the other's behavior and the impact it had:
- The Inner Critic/Coach describes the frustration or concern it felt when the Escaper/Inner Nurturer disengaged and avoided challenges. It can express how this instigated its critical behaviors in an effort to regain control.
- The Escaper/Inner Nurturer shares how it felt in response to the Inner Critic/Coach's judgment—overwhelmed, discouraged or shut down—and how that led to further withdrawal.

Both Parts Apologize and Commit to New Roles: After listening to each other, both parts have the chance to take responsibility and commit to a healthier relationship:
- The Inner Critic/Coach offers an apology for its past critical and judgmental behavior. It explains its new role as a source of encouragement, constructive feedback and motivation rather than harsh criticism.
- The Escaper/Inner Nurturer offers an apology for its avoidance patterns, clarifying that they were meant to offer protection but may have come across as disengagement. It explains how it is now committed to offering true self-care, emotional support and presence instead of escaping.

Define a New Collaboration: With these acknowledgments in place, both parts discuss how they can work together as a team moving forward.
- How can the Inner Critic/Coach offer feedback and encouragement without avoidance?
- How can the Escaper/Inner Nurturer stay engaged while providing care and support?
- What strategies can they use to maintain a balanced and respectful relationship?
- Do they have any requests or boundaries to help ensure they don't instigate each other in the future?

Close the Process: Thank both parts for showing up in this process. Invite them to acknowledge each other in a closing gesture that feels right—this could be a verbal thank you, a handshake, a bow, a hug, a nod or even a small movement like a dance or placing a hand over the heart. Offer any parting words that bring closure and reinforce the shift toward a more relational and supportive connection.

Collective Unburdening: Transforming the Inner Critic, Shame and the Escaper

In this process, you'll guide the Inner Critic, Shame and the Escaper through a collective unburdening and transformation. This threshold ceremony allows them to release their old patterns and embrace their new, healthier roles as the Inner Coach, the unburdened Raw Experience and the Inner Nurturer. This marks their commitment to a more harmonious and supportive internal system.

Ground in Self-Energy: Begin by grounding yourself in Self-energy. Take deep breaths, centering yourself in calm, openness and curiosity. Allow a sense of loving presence to arise within you, creating a stable foundation for this process.

Invite the Parts Forward: Call forth the Inner Critic, Shame and the Escaper to step into awareness. Assure them that this is a safe space for transformation and that they will be supported throughout the process.

Create a Safe Space: Visualize a safe space where this unburdening will take place. It could be a natural setting, a serene room or anywhere that feels secure and inviting. Set the intention for this ceremony as one of healing, release and transformation, affirming that each part will be honored and respected.

Acknowledge Old Patterns: Give each part a chance to express how it has been operating in its old role:
- The Inner Critic reflects on its history of judgment and control, acknowledging how it impacted both the Escaper and Shame. It expresses its readiness to release these old patterns.
- Shame shares how it has been affected by the Inner Critic's harshness and the Escaper's avoidance. It speaks to the weight of the stories of unworthiness and deficiency it has carried and expresses its readiness to let them go.
- The Escaper reflects on how it has used avoidance to cope with difficult emotions, recognizing the unintended harm of turning away instead of facing feelings. It expresses its readiness to embrace a new way of being.

Express Gratitude for Past Roles: From the stance of Self, express appreciation for each part's positive intentions—even though their strategies caused harm, they were all trying to protect you in their own way. Express how necessary and even lifesaving some of these strategies might have been.

Pass Through the Threshold of Transformation: Now, each part will pass through a symbolic threshold—marking the release of its old role and the emergence of something new. Invite your parts to choose what kind of threshold they'll cross:

a doorway, an archway, a bridge, a curtain of mist or anything else that feels meaningful. As each part approaches, guide it to recognize that it no longer has to carry out its old, burdened role. Just before or as it passes through the threshold, have it lay down that role—perhaps placing it at the edge or allowing it to dissolve in the moment of crossing. You might visualize fire, water, wind or earth carrying the old energy away, leaving the part lighter and freer. Then, one by one, invite each part to step through the threshold and emerge in its new form:

- See the Inner Critic releasing its harshness and stepping forward as the Inner Coach, a part that offers support, encouragement and clarity without judgment.
- See Shame shedding its old stories and emerging unburdened as Raw Experience, now embodying self-acceptance, dignity and emotional truth.
- See the Escaper letting go of avoidance and stepping through as the Inner Nurturer, a part that offers grounding, comfort and care in the face of discomfort.

Welcome the New Roles: Now, introduce these transformed parts to one another in their new forms. Affirm their new roles and how they can now work together as a collaborative, supportive team. Allow them to express their commitment to this new way of being and to supporting one another in a more balanced and harmonious internal system.

Create a Symbol of Unity: Visualize a symbol that represents the unity of your newly transformed parts. This could be a radiant triangle, a glowing heart or a beam of interwoven light—something that embodies wholeness and internal harmony. See this symbol radiating warmth and energy, and allow your Inner Coach, Raw Experience and Inner Nurturer to absorb this light.
- The Inner Coach is filled with clarity and encouragement.
- The Raw Experience receives compassion and self-acceptance.
- The Inner Nurturer receives strength and support.

Let this image serve as a reminder that these parts are now working together. You can return to this symbol whenever you need to reconnect with their balanced, aligned presence.

Close the Ceremony: Offer gratitude to your parts for their willingness to evolve and for the gifts they now offer: wisdom, self-love and inner strength. Express appreciation in a way that feels right—this could be a spoken thank you, a bow, an embrace, a moment of stillness or any other closing gesture. Visualize the sacred space gently fading, leaving you feeling grounded, whole and deeply connected to your Self-energy. Take a few moments to integrate this experience, noticing any shifts in how you feel and how these parts now interact with one another.

Create Your Own Ritual

Beyond the guided exercises, you can design your own rituals or symbolic practices to represent your transformation. Expressing this journey in a personal and creative way can deepen your connection to the process, making it more tangible and meaningful. You might draw or paint your evolution from the Shame Triangle to the Self-Love Triangle, visually capturing how each part has changed. One of Jessica's clients, an avid quilter, created a symbolic quilt, with each patch representing a step in their journey.

Other creative expressions could include:
- Writing poetry or personal narratives that tell the story of transforming your Shame Triangle
- Composing music or creating a playlist that reflects your emotional journey
- Choreographing a dance or movement piece that embodies the transformation of your parts
- Using origami, jewelry, paint or sculpture to represent your parts and their evolution

- Building an altar with meaningful objects, natural elements or candles to symbolize your shift
- Planting a garden or tending to a specific plant as a living metaphor for growth and renewal
- Recording an audio message to your parts—or from them—to mark the shift in your relationship
- Creating a ritual with water (a bath, a river, rain) to release the past and invite what's next

Whatever form it takes, creating a personal ritual offers a concrete way to honor your work. It helps mark the shift that's taken place, so the transformation becomes something you can return to, remember and carry forward.

CONCLUSION

As this book draws to a close, we hope you understand that no matter how deep your struggles have felt—no matter how messy, tangled or overwhelming your patterns may seem—you are not beyond change. Even if you have been broken, you are not beyond repair.

By now, you should have a clear sense that the parts of you that once felt like burdens—your self-doubt, your fears, your perfectionism, your avoidance—were never flaws. They were signs of your adaptability, shaped by what you needed to get through a specific situation or time. These strategies helped you survive. But now, they need to be updated to support the life you're living and actively creating. You and your parts are not problems to be solved. They are patterns to understand and relationships to shift. When met with Self, even the most entrenched parts can change. You are a living, breathing process—a story still unfolding, a body still learning its own rhythms, a heart still opening to what it needs and a mind still learning how to see clearly.

The Shame Triangle has a way of convincing us that damage is permanent, that the ways we have fractured under the weight of our pain make us unworthy, unfixable. But breaking is not the same as ending. In Japan, there is an ancient practice called *kintsugi*, the art of repairing broken pottery with gold. Instead of trying to hide the cracks, *kintsugi* highlights them by filling each fracture with shimmering veins of lacquer mixed with powdered gold, silver or platinum. Something that was once shattered, sharp-edged and nonfunctional is made whole again—not in spite of its brokenness, but because of it. The scars become part of its beauty, a testament to its history rather than a flaw to be erased.

Nature teaches us this same lesson: Regeneration is always possible.

When a wildfire tears through a forest, our human eyes see destruction. We see loss—the towering trees reduced to skeletal remains, structures gone, the ground covered in ash, the silence where leaves once rustled and birds sang. But the forest has a different experience. It does not see fire as the end. It knows something we don't.

The fire clears out what is overgrown, making space for new life. It releases nutrients, enriching the soil in a way that nothing else can. And some trees can only grow after a fire—heat cracks open their cones, releasing the seeds locked inside. Without the fire, they would have remained sealed inside, dormant, never able to sprout. What looks like devastation to us is, to the forest, a necessary stage of renewal. The old must burn away to make space for something new.

We, Dave and Jessica, saw a similar form of regeneration firsthand in the aftermath of Hurricane Helene in Asheville, North Carolina. The storm carved through the land with devastating force. Buildings, homes and entire streets were washed away by the floods. Millions of trees were knocked down, their roots exposed like open wounds. Some of what was destroyed will never return to what it was before. Some things are lost forever.

And yet, even in the wake of such destruction, the land is rebuilding itself. The forest, in many ways, is fine. The fallen trees are not just debris—they have become the foundation for new growth. Disintegrating into the soil, they provide the nourishment that allows new saplings to rise. What looked like an ending was, in many ways, just another stage in the cycle of renewal.

You are nature. And this ability is part of you, too.

The Shame Triangle—its rigid roles, its heavy burdens—is not a life sentence. It is a pattern, and all patterns can be reshaped.

In reading these pages, in reflecting on your own experience, in even the smallest shifts in how you relate to yourself, you have already begun that work. Right now, in real time, you are regrowing.

Change does not happen in a single step or way. It happens in big leaps and in slow, steady movements. It happens in the chaos of massive storms that knock us down, in the two-steps-forward, three-steps-back rhythm of trial and error, and in the quiet, almost imperceptible shifts that accumulate over time. It happens in ways that feel sudden, in ways that feel frustratingly slow and in ways that don't feel like change at all—until one day, you look back and realize you are standing in an entirely different place. Trust in your process, whatever its pace may be.

Being Self-centered is not about living without challenges. It is not about reaching some final state of enlightenment where you never struggle again. It is about being more centered, attuned and willing to navigate. It is about knowing how to shift between expansion and contraction, energy and rest, engagement and retreat, without losing yourself to the extremes.

When the Inner Critic transforms into the Inner Coach, discipline is no longer punishment—it is a practice of values-based encouragement. Accountability is infused with kindness. Mistakes become learning, not proof of failure. When Shame shifts into Raw Experience, you no longer shrink, resist or try to conceal what arises. You allow it to be present. When the Escaper evolves into the Inner Nurturer, self-care becomes devotion, rather than avoidance. Instead of pushing yourself to exhaustion, proving your worth through effort, you embrace rest as a necessity, not a luxury. Instead of disconnecting, you turn toward yourself, learning to meet what you once tried to outrun.

Living in the Self-Love Triangle is about remembering who you are beneath the layers of old stories. It is about making space for all of you: the parts that are still learning, the parts that are still afraid, the parts that are finally beginning to trust.

Let the work you've done here be your guide. Stay with this process. Keep applying what you've learned. Keep turning toward yourself. Keep honoring the shifts, big and small. Keep going. It's worth it, and so are you!

∆

APPENDIX

EASE Process for Working with Your Parts

This exercise comes from our book *Polywise* and is included in this appendix so you can continue working with your parts after completing the Self LOVE U process. While the Self LOVE U framework helped you build an initial connection with your inner world, this exercise offers a simple way to continue to dialogue with your parts.

- E   Externalize
- A   Ask
- S   Soothe
- E   Educate or Emancipate

Before you begin, turn inward and center into Self for several breaths.

E   Externalize Your Part

Just as you located a part in the Self LOVE U process, begin by identifying the Shame Triangle part you want to work with. Imagine that this part is outside of your body, positioned directly in front of you. Take a moment to feel this part outside of you.

A   Ask

Once the part is externalized, ask it about its experience. What is it struggling with? What feelings or needs are coming up for it?

Since you are working with the Shame Triangle parts, tailor your questions to their specific concerns:
- **Inner Critic:** What are you afraid will happen if you stop being critical?
- **Shame:** What pain or fear are you carrying? What are you trying to protect me from?
- **Escaper:** What discomfort are you trying to avoid? What do you fear would happen if you stayed present?

Ask with genuine curiosity. Let your part express its concerns, fears or hesitations without judgment.

S   Soothe

Once you understand the part's feelings and needs, soothe it with validation and empathy. Acknowledge its fears and let it know it makes sense that it feels this way.

Soothing can take different forms:
- Speaking gently and offering reassurance
- Imagining sitting beside the part, offering comfort
- Visualizing holding it in a warm embrace or offering a gentle touch

As you soothe, imagine your part truly receiving your care. Let it settle, relax and release any tension it's holding. Stay with this step until you notice a shift—a softening, a lightness or a sense of relief.

E   Educate or Emancipate

Once your part feels soothed, it is ready to be educated or even emancipated.
- **Educate:** Remind the part of the updates from the Self LOVE U process. Let it know that you are no longer living in the past, that your circumstances have changed and that you now have the ability to meet your needs in new, healthier ways. Encourage it to release survival mode and step into a role that supports growth and well-being.

If this part still feels uncertain, reassure it by describing the supportive roles of the Self-Love Triangle. Help it understand that it can contribute in ways that are empowering rather than critical, fearful or avoidant.
- **Emancipate:** If the part no longer wishes to hold onto its old responsibilities, let it know that it is free. It does not have to take on a new job if it doesn't want one. Instead, it can simply exist—resting, playing, creating, exploring or just being. Some parts may transform into a sense of lightness, curiosity or even joy. Others may prefer to fade into the background, no longer needing to hold a defined role. Trust the part to know what feels right, and honor whatever choice it makes.

Close the Practice

Take a moment to breathe and integrate this shift. Thank the part for its willingness to release what no longer serves you and embrace new possibilities. When you feel ready, gently bring your awareness back to the present moment.

REFERENCES

Arenander, A., and F. T. Travis. 2004. *Brain Patterns of Self-Awareness* [Research report]. Brain Research Institute. https://brainresearchinstitute.org/brain-patterns-of-self-awareness.pdf.

Bowen, M. 1978. *Family Therapy in Clinical Practice.* Jason Aronson.

Brach, T. 2003. *Radical Acceptance: Embracing Your Life with the Heart of a Buddha.* Bantam Books.

Brave Heart, M. Y. H. 2000. "Wakiksuyapi: Carrying the Historical Trauma of the Lakota." *Tulane Studies in Social Welfare* 21–22: 245–66.

Breslau, N., G. C. Davis, P. Andreski, and E. L. Peterson. 1991. "Traumatic Events and Post-Traumatic Stress Disorder in an Urban Population of Young Adults." *Archives of General Psychiatry* 48 (3): 216–22. https://doi.org/10.1001/archpsyc.1991.01810270028003.

Brown, B. 2012. *Daring Greatly: How the Courage to Be Vulnerable Transforms the Way We Live, Love, Parent, and Lead.* Penguin.

Brown, R. P., and P. L. Gerbarg. 2012. *The Healing Power of the Breath: Simple Techniques to Reduce Stress and Anxiety, Enhance Concentration, and Balance Your Emotions.* Shambhala Publications.

Campbell, J. (1949) 2008. *The Hero with a Thousand Faces.* 3rd ed. New World Library.

Cwinn, E. 2018. *Self-Criticism and Responses to Self-Critical Statements: An Investigation of Self-Criticism, Self-Submission, Self-Compassion, and Attack-Resistance.* University of Guelph.

Dweck, C. S. 2006. *Mindset: The New Psychology of Success*. Random House.

Fern, J. 2020. *Polysecure: Attachment, Trauma and Consensual Nonmonogamy*. Thornapple Press.

Fern, J., and D. Cooley. 2023. *Polywise: A Deeper Dive into Navigating Open Relationships*. Thornapple Press.

Gilligan, C. 1982. *In a Different Voice: Psychological Theory and Women's Development*. Harvard University Press.

Halamová, J., J. Koróniová, M. Kanovský, M. Kénesy Túniyová and N. Kupeli. 2019. "Psychological and Physiological Effects of Emotion-Focused Training for Self-Compassion and Self-Protection." *Research in Psychotherapy: Psychopathology, Process and Outcome*, 22 (2): 265–280. https://doi.org/10.4081/ripppo.2019.358.

Hirschberger, G. 2018. "Collective Trauma and the Social Construction of Meaning." *Frontiers in Psychology* 9: 1441. https://doi.org/10.3389/fpsyg.2018.01441.

Johnston, A. 2000. *Eating in the Light of the Moon: How Women Can Transform Their Relationship with Food Through Myths, Metaphors, and Storytelling*. Gürze Books.

Kaufman, G. 1989. *The Psychology of Shame: Theory and Treatment of Shame-Based Syndromes*. Springer.

Lee, D. A. 2005. "The Perfect Nurturer: A Model to Develop a Compassionate Mind within the Context of Cognitive Therapy." In *Compassion: Conceptualisations, Research and Use in Psychotherapy*, edited by P. Gilbert. Routledge.

Levine, P. A. 1997. *Waking the Tiger: Healing Trauma*. North Atlantic Books.

Levine, P. A. 2010. *In an Unspoken Voice: How the Body Releases Trauma and Restores Goodness*. North Atlantic Books.

Maté, G. 2003. *When the Body Says No: Understanding the Stress-Disease Connection*. Wiley.

Maté, G. 2010. *In the Realm of Hungry Ghosts: Close Encounters with Addiction*. North Atlantic Books.

Neff, K. D. 2003. "Self-Compassion: An Alternative Conceptualization of a Healthy Attitude Toward Oneself." *Self and Identity* 2 (2): 85–101. https://doi.org/10.1080/15298860309032.

Neff, K. D. 2021. *Fierce Self-Compassion: How Women Can Harness Kindness to Speak Up, Claim Their Power, and Thrive*. HarperWave.

Ogden, P., K. Minton, and C. Pain. 2006. *Trauma and the Body: A Sensorimotor Approach to Psychotherapy*. W.W. Norton & Company.

Porges, S. W. 2003. "The Polyvagal Theory: Phylogenetic Contributions to Social Behavior." *Physiology & Behavior* 79 (3): 503–13. https://doi.org/10.1016/S0031-9384(03)00156-2

Porges, S. W. 2011. *The Polyvagal Theory: Neurophysiological Foundations of Emotions, Attachment, Communication, and Self-Regulation*. Norton & Company.

Ranke, K. 1981. "Problems of Categories in Folk Prose." Translated by C. Lindahl. *Folklore Forum* 14 (1): 1–17.

Rocha, L. F., and M. A. Penido. 2024. "Compassion-Focused Therapy: A Transdiagnostic Approach to Self-Criticism in Clinical Practice." In *Transdiagnostic Approaches in Cognitive Behavioral Therapy*, edited by A. C. Ornelas. Springer.

Roelofs, K. 2017. "Freeze for Action: Neurobiological Mechanisms in Animal and Human Freezing." *Philosophical Transactions of the Royal Society B: Biological Sciences* 372 (1718): 20160206. https://doi.org/10.1098/rstb.2016.0206.

Roelofs, K., M. A. Hagenaars and J. F. Stins (2010). Facing freeze: Social threat induces bodily freeze in humans. *Psychological Science*, 21(11), 1575–1581. https://doi.org/10.1177/0956797610384746.

Rothschild, B. 2000. *The Body Remembers: The Psychophysiology of Trauma and Trauma Treatment*. W.W. Norton & Company.

Schauer, M., F. Neuner, and T. Elbert. 2011. *Narrative Exposure Therapy: A Short-Term Treatment for Traumatic Stress Disorders*. Hogrefe Publishing.

Schwartz, R. C. 1995. *Internal Family Systems Therapy*. Guilford Press.

Schwartz, R. C. 2021. *No Bad Parts: Healing Trauma and Restoring Wholeness with the Internal Family Systems Model.* Sounds True.

Schwartz, R. C., and M. Sweezy. 2020. *Internal Family Systems Therapy.* 2nd ed. The Guilford Press.

Sinko, A. L. 2017. "Legacy Burdens." In *Innovations and Elaborations in Internal Family Systems Therapy*, edited by M. Sweezy and E. L. Ziskind. Routledge.

Sovik, R. 2000. "The Science of Breathing—The Yogic View." *Progress in Brain Research* 122: 491–505.

Suzuki, S. 1970. *Zen Mind, Beginner's Mind.* Shambhala.

Vago, D. R., and D. A. Silbersweig. 2012. "Self-Awareness, Self-Regulation, and Self-Transcendence (S-ART): A Framework for Understanding the Neurobiological Mechanisms of Mindfulness." *Frontiers in Human Neuroscience* 6 (296). https://doi.org/10.3389/fnhum.2012.00296.

Van der Kolk, B. 2014. *The Body Keeps the Score: Brain, Mind, and Body in the Healing of Trauma.* Viking.

Walker, P. 2013. *Complex PTSD: From Surviving to Thriving.* Azure Coyote.

Weiss, B. L. 1988. *Many Lives, Many Masters: The True Story of a Prominent Psychiatrist, His Young Patient, and the Past-Life Therapy That Changed Both Their Lives.* Simon & Schuster.

White, M., and D. Epston. 1990. *Narrative Means to Therapeutic Ends.* Norton.

Wolynn, M. 2016. *It Didn't Start with You: How Inherited Family Trauma Shapes Who We Are and How to End the Cycle.* Penguin Books.

Yehuda, R., N. P. Daskalakis, L. M. Bierer, H. N. Bader, T. Klengel, F. Holsboer and E. B. Binder. 2016. "Holocaust Exposure Induced Intergenerational Effects on FKBP5 Methylation." *Biological Psychiatry* 80 (5): 372–80.

Yehuda, R., and A. Lehrner. 2018. "Intergenerational Transmission of Trauma Effects: Putative Role of Epigenetic Mechanisms." *World Psychiatry* 17 (3): 243–57. https://doi.org/10.1002/wps.20568.

Zehr, H. 1990. *Changing Lenses: A New Focus for Crime and Justice.* Herald Press.

INDEX

Page numbers in bold represent tables and diagrams.

4-4-4-4 breathing, 221–2
5-4-3-2-1 grounding exercise, 221

ableism, 103
absent but implicit, 179–83
academic pressures, 106
adversarial mindset, 256–8, 262–3, **264**
ageism, 103
aggression, 22, 238
ancestral trauma, 281
anchor stance exercise, 226–7
the Anima and Animus, 6–7
archetypal patterns, 7
archetypal roles. *See* Drama Triangle
assertiveness, 62
Attuned Supporter, 63–4
awake awareness exercise, 135–6

ball of beliefs exercise, 274–6
beauty standards, 105–6
beginner's mindset, **264, 265**, 269–71, 273
binary mindset, 258–9, 262–4, **264**, 267
body, 3, 152–60, 169–71, 174–6. *See also* Four F responses; Shame Triangle and body
body image, 105–6
body wisdom, 229–32
boundary-setting exercise, 226–7
box breathing (4-4-4-4) exercise, 221–2
Brach, Tara, 82
Breath of Fire (Kapalabhati) exercise, 224–5
Brown, Brené, 81
Buddhism, 13–15
burdens, 181–2

calm, 124, 144. *See also* Eight C's of Self
Campbell, Joseph, 51
capitalist ideologies, 101–2
CARE exercise for feelings as inside, 246–7
CARE exercise for feelings as parts, 245–6
cause/contribute/condone, 61
chairwork dialogue exercise, 145–6
cisnormativity, 104–5
clarity, 124, 144. *See also* Eight C's of Self
classism, 105
collective ancestral unburdening exercise, 295–7
collective trauma, 282
collective unburdening exercises, 313–16
colonialism legacies, 102
compassion, 124, 143. *See also* Eight C's of Self
confidence, 124, 144. *See also* Eight C's of Self
conflict, 45–7, 52, 129
connectedness, 124, 144–5. *See also* Eight C's of Self
Conscious Participant, 63
consumerism, 106–7

Cooley, David, 30–1, 71–2, 238–41, 305–6
cord cutting exercise, 290–2
courage, 124, 144. *See also* Eight C's of Self
creativity, 124, 145. *See also* Eight C's of Self
cultural appropriation, 14
curiosity, 124, 143. *See also* Eight C's of Self

defensiveness, 129, 130, 162
Descartes, René, 3
dialogue with parts
  about, 177
  concerns about, 183–6
  Escapers, 202–7
  Inner Critic, 187–95
  process of, 186–7
  Shame, 195–202
  See also Restorative Relationship Conversation model
double listening, 180–3
drama, 7, **8**
Drama Triangle
  about, **8**, 8–9, 20, **21**, 39–40, 42–3
  cause/contribute/condone, 61
  getting off of, 56–65
  impacts, 59
  intentions for future, 61–2
  payoffs, 48, **49**
  role preference, 58
  self-accountability, 60–4
  self-awareness, 56–9
  self-regulation, 59–60
  Shame and, 80–1
  starting, 53–4
  storytelling and, 50–1
  stress response system and, 51–3
  switching positions in, 40–2
  triggers, 59
  victim consciousness, 43–4
Dweck, Carol, 259–60, 268

Earley, Jay, 17
EASE exercise, 188, 323–4
Eastern philosophy, 13–14
Eating in the Light of the Moon (Johnston), 202–3
ecstatic shaking exercise, 219–20
educate inner part, 191–2, 205–6. *See also* Self LOVE U
Eight C's of Self, 124–5, 127, 143–5
embracing inner part, 200. *See also* Self LOVE U
epigenetic healing, 289
epigenetic inheritance, 282
Epston, David, 10
Escapers
  ableism and, 103
  about, 5, 88–93
  ageism and, 103
  beauty standards and, 106
  body and, 157, 159–60
  capitalist ideologies and, 102
  classism and, 105
  colonialism/slavery and, 102
  consumerism and, 107
  externalization, 96–7
  Four F responses and, 215–16
  gender and sexuality, 104
  heart and, 163
  individualism and, 103
  Inner Critic and, 88, 89, 93
  instant gratification culture and, 108
  mapping effects of, 93–5
  mind and, 167
  patriarchy and, 103
  perfectionism, 23
  positive events and, 115–16
  power over, 95–6
  professional pressure, 106
  Raw Experience and, 202
  self-love and, 27
  Shame and, 88, 90, 97–8, 215
  Shame Triangle and, **21**, 21–2, 24

shift to Inner Nurturer, **28**
substance use culture, 107–8
taking in/taking a stand, 95
transforming, 177, 202–7
See also Restorative
 Relationship Conversation
 model; Shame Triangle
everything out of the room!
 exercise, 227–9
exercises overview, 33
Exiles, 23–4
expert mindset, 261–2,
 262–4, **265**, 269–70
externalization
 about, 11–12
 Escapers, 96–7, 104
 Inner Critic, 77–8
 Shame, 86–7, 198
external triggers, 111–12
external validation, 132–3
eye-tracking exercise, 222–3

family constellations work, 287–8
Fern, Jessica
 about, 29–30
 diverse cultures and, 12–13
 Drama Triangle and, 41–2
 Eastern philosophy, 13–14
 Escapers and, 92–3
 IFS and, 16–19
 inherited Shame Triangle, 284–6
 Inner Critic and, 284–6
 journey to parts work, 6–12
 love and, 234–7
 positive events and, 114–16
 the Self and, 119–21
 Shame and, 91–2
 Universal Me meditation
  exercise, 137
Firefighters, 23–4
fixed mindset, 259–60,
 262–4, **265**, 268

Four F responses
 about, 210–11
 Escapers and, 215–16
 Inner Critic and, 211–13
 regulating fawn response, 226–9
 regulating fight response, 218–20
 regulating flight response, 221–3
 regulating freeze response, 223–6
 Shame and, 213–14
Freud, Sigmund, 6

gender and sexuality, 104–5, 113
generational healing, 289
gentle rocking exercise, 224
grounding push, 219
growth mindset, **264**,
 265, 268–9, 273

heart
 about, 152–5, 160–5, 254
 centering exercises, 244–54
 as courageous, 254
 integration and reflection, 174–6
 self-evaluation, 171–3
Hellinger, Bert, 287–8
heteronormativity, 104–5
historical trauma, 282
humming exercise, 224

individualism, 103
injustice, 181
inner abuser, 70–1
Inner Coach
 about, 321
 body and, 159
 exercises for, 308–9, 311–13
 heart and, 164
 mind and, 168
 reminding Inner Critic of, 193–4
 Self LOVE U, 188–9
 shift to, 27, **28**
 See also Self-Love Triangle

Inner Critic
  ableism and, 103
  about, 4, 19–20, 68–73
  ageism and, 103
  beauty standards and, 105–6
  body and, 157, 159
  capitalist ideologies and, 102
  classism and, 105
  colonialism/slavery and, 102
  consumerism and, 107
  Escapers and, 88, 89, 93
  externalization, 77–8
  Fern and, 81, 284–6
  fight response and, 211–13
  gender and sexuality, 104
  heart and, 162–3
  individualism and, 103
  instant gratification culture and, 108
  as Manager, 24
  mapping effects of, 73–4
  mind and, 166–7
  patriarchy and, 104
  positive events and, 114, 115
  power over, 76–7
  professional pressure, 106
  self-care and, 27
  Shame and, 21, 78, 97
  Shame Triangle and, 21
  shift to Inner Coach, 27, **28**, 29
  substance use culture, 107–8
  taking in/taking a stand, 76
  transforming, 177, 187–95, 193–4
  triggers, 111
  See also Inner Coach; Restorative Relationship Conversation model; Shame Triangle
Inner Nurturers
  about, 321
  body and, 159
  exercises for, 310–15
  heart and, 164–5
  mind and, 169
  shift to, **28**

inner parts
  about, 2–4
  accomplishments and, 127–8
  connecting to, 141
  as guided by Self, 131
  healing, 130
  perceiving, 17–18
  Self-energy and, 127
  as shaped by role, 128
  skills dealing with, 150–1
  speaking from/for, 128–30, **132**, 145–7
  See also Internal Family Systems
instant gratification culture, 108
integration and reflection, 174–5
intergenerational trauma, 282
Internal Family Systems (IFS)
  about, 16–17
  dialogue with parts, 184
  legacy unburdening exercise, 292–4
  the Self in, 123–4
  Self-leadership, 126
  versus Shame Triangle, 23–4
internal triggers, 112–13
internalization
  colonialism/slavery, 102
  consumerism, 106–7
  gender and sexuality, 104–5
  harsh judgments, 48
  Inner Critic and, 72
  narrative theory and, 9–10, 11
  professional pressure, 106
  recognizing, 108–9
  Shame and, 78

Johnston, Anita, 202–3
journaling from part exercise, 147–8
journaling from Self exercise, 146–7
Jung, Carl, 6–7

Karpman, Stephen, 7, 45

legacy burdens, 282
legacy unburdening exercise, 288, 292–4
Levine, Peter, 288
liberation, 37–8
locate inner part. *See* Self LOVE U
love, 165, 233–8

Managers, 23–4
meeting ancestors exercise, 302–3
mind, 3, 152–5, 165–9, 173–6. *See also* Shame Triangle and mind
Mindset (Dweck), 268
Myss, Caroline, 7

narcissism, 79–80
narrative theory, 9–11, 50
nervous system regulation, 150
"no" practice exercise, 226–7
non-dual mindset, 223–4, 263–4, **264, 265**, 267–8, 273

orienting response reset exercise, 222–3
origin story. *See* Self LOVE U
origins of Shame Triangle, 99–100
Outer Critic, 22

past life trauma, 282
patriarchy, 103–4
perfectionism, 21, 23, 102, 106
performance, 101–2
the Persecutor
about, **8, 21**, 39
awareness of role, 58
costs to self/others, **49**
fight response, 52
payoffs, **49**
roles/beliefs, **55**
shift to assertiveness, 62
start of Drama Triangle and, 53–4
victim consciousness and, 44
See also Drama Triangle

the Persona, 6–7
physical limitations, 158–9
pillow punching exercise, 220
Plato, 3
Polysecure (Fern), 30
Polywise (Fern), 30, 188, 228
positive events, 113–14
poststructuralism, 9–10
preferred beliefs exercise, 279–80
primal roar exercise, 220
problem-saturated story, 10
professional pressure, 106
protection
  Escapers and, 92–3, 203, 215–16
  Shame and, 196–7
  updating, 249–51
punishment, 47–8

Ranke, Kurt, 50
Raw Experience
  about, 178, 321
  avoidance and, 202
  exercises for, 309–11, 313–16
  updating Shame, 201
  See also Self-Love Triangle
regeneration, 319–20
regret, 69. *See also* Inner Critic
relationships, 75, 80, 85–6
religious doctrines, 101
the Rescuer
  about, **8, 21**, 39
  awareness of role, 58
  costs to self/others, **49**
  fawn response, 52
  flight response, 52
  payoffs, **49**
  roles/beliefs, **55**
  shift to Attuned Supporter, 63–4
  start of Drama Triangle and, 53–4
  victim consciousness and, 43–44
  as victimized, 54
  See also Drama Triangle

restorative justice, 31–2. *See also* Restorative Relationship Conversation model
restorative mindset, 263, **265**, 265–6, 273
restorative paradigm, 265–6
Restorative Relationship Conversation (RRC) model, 32, 305–7. *See also* Self-Love Triangle
righteous Victim, 44
risk assessment, 69–70
rituals, 289, 316–17
root down exercise, 277–9
R's of releasing beliefs, 274–80

Schwartz, Richard, 16, 33, 123–4. *See also* Internal Family Systems
the Self
  about, 16–17, 148
  as being, 128
  as detached, 148
  as elusive, 149–50
  Fern and, 119–21
  as guiding parts, 131
  in IFS, 123–4
  journaling exercise, 146–7
  metaphors for, 150
  Self-energy and, 121–3
  as witness, 118
  See also Self LOVE U
self-accountability, 60–4
self-awareness, 56–9, 121
self-care, 27
Self-centered model
  about, 151–2, 321
  body, 155–60, 169–71, 174–6
  evaluating three centers, 169–74
  heart, 160–5, 171–3, 174–6, 255–6
  integration and reflection, 174–5
  mind, 165–9, 173–6
  Self-leadership and, 154
self-compassion, 27

Self-connection exercises
  about, 134, 148
  awake awareness beyond identities, 135–6
  chairwork dialogue exercise, 145–6
  Eight C's of Self, 143–5
  journaling from part, 147–8
  journaling from Self, 146–7
self-defeat, 259–60
Self-energy
  about, 127
  Eight C's of Self and, 124–5
  to Self connect, 16, 188–9, 197, 203–4
  Self-Love Triangle, 28
self-evaluation, 169–74
Self-leadership
  about, **126**
  body and, 153–4, 158, 159
  challenging source of meaning, 132–3
  complexity of inner world and, 128
  heart and, 153–4, 160, 163
  mind and, 153–4, 167
  mindset prompts, 271–4
  mindsets, 262–3, 263–71
  Self-centered and, 154
  Self-Love Triangle and, 28
  transformation and, 26–7
  as way of being, 19
self-love, 27
Self-Love Triangle
  about, **28**, 321–2
  exercises for, 308–17
  integrity, 185
  RRC and, 305–6
  self-reflection, 185
  shift to, 27–8
  See also transformation
Self LOVE U, 188–9, 197–202
self-regulation, 59–60
Self-Therapy (Earley), 17

sexuality, 104–5, 113
the Shadow, 6–7
shamanic practices, 14–15, 288
shame
  about, 5
  defined, 35
  fear and, 35
  Fern and, 81
  inner critic shape-shifting and, 20
  in interwoven system, 22–3
  mental health and, 168
Shame
  ableism and, 103
  about, 5, 78–83
  beauty standards and, 105
  body and, 157, 159
  colonialism/slavery and, 102
  defined, 35
  Escapers and, 80, 88, 90, 97–8, 215
  Exiles and, 24
  freeze response and, 213–14
  heart and, 163, 164
  inadequacy and, 183
  Inner Critic and, 21, 22, 22–3, 78, 97
  mapping effects of, 83–4
  mind and, 167, 168
  pain as overwhelming, 196
  positive events and, 114–15
  as protector, 196–7
  self-compassion and, 27
  shift to Raw Experience, **28**
  struggle and, 108
  taking it in/taking a stand, 86–7
  transforming, 177–8, 195–202
  the Victim and, 80–1
  wounds and, 182, 196–7, 198–9
  See also Raw Experience; Restorative Relationship Conversation model; Shame Triangle
Shame Triangle
  about, 4–5, 25–6, 319–21
  distortion and, 82
  fixed mindset, 268
  versus IFS, 23–5
  inherited, 281–2, 286–7, 289–304
  Inner Critic and, **21**, 21–3
  interaction of roles, 97–8
  as internal enforcer, 22
  multiple versions of, 67–8
  needing, 184–5
  nervous system and (*see* Shame Triangle and body)
  origins, 99–108
  positive events and, 113–14
  reinforcement of, 117–18
  Self-energy and, 122
  shift to Self-Love Triangle, 27–9, **28**
  triggers, 110–13
  See also Escapers; Inner Critic; Self-Love Triangle; Shame
Shame Triangle and body
  about, 209–10
  nervous system responses overview, 210–11
  regulating fawn response, 226–9
  regulating fight response, 218–20
  regulating flight response, 221–3
  regulating freeze response, 223–6
Shame Triangle and heart
  about, 233–4
  armor and love, 234–44
  heart center exercises, 244–54
Shame Triangle and mind
  about, 255–6
  adversarial mindset, 256–8, 262–3, **265**, 273
  binary mindset, 258–9, 262–4, **265**, 267, 273
  expert mindset, 261–2, 262–4, **265**, 269–70, 273
  fixed mindset, 259–60, 262–4, **265**, 273
  Self-led mindset exercises, 274–80

Shame Triangle and mind *(continued)*
　Self-led mindset prompts, 271–3
　Self-led mindsets, 262–3,
　　263–71, **264–5**
Shoshin, 269
Sinko, Anne, 292–4
slavery legacies, 102
social media, 43, 111
solo family constellation
　exercise, 298–9
somatic exercise, 299–302
somatic experiencing, 288
spirituality, 13–15, 125
spoken "no" practice exercise, 226–7
storytelling, 50–1
stress response system, 51–3
substance use culture, 107–8
survival mechanisms, 52–3, 210–11
Suzuki, Shunryu, 269
systemic constellations, 288

transformation
　about, 185, 186–7
　accountability and, 185
　Escapers, 177, 202–7 *(see also* Inner Nurturers)
　Inner Critic, 177, 187–95, 193–4 *(see also* Inner Coach)
　as process, 35
　retirement, 186
　Self-leadership and, 26–7
　Shame, 177–8, 195–202 *(see also* Raw Experience)
translation, Inner Critic and, 194–5
trauma
　Cooley and, 239
　Drama Triangle and, 45–6
　exercises for, 289–303
　inherited, 281–9
　open heart and, 237
　Self-regulation and, 151
trauma-informed care, 31–2
triggers, 110–13

truth, 129, 130, 271–2

unburdening, 288, 292–7, 313–16
Universal Me meditation
　exercise, 136–9
unworthiness, 182
update inner part. *See* Self LOVE U

vagal toning exercise, 224
validation of inner part.
　See Self LOVE U
the Victim
　about, **8, 21,** 39
　awareness of role, 58
　costs to self/others, **49**
　fawn response, 52
　flight response, 52
　freeze response, 52
　payoffs, **49**
　as righteous, 44
　roles/beliefs, **55**
　Shame and, 80–1
　shift to Conscious Participant, 63
　start of Drama Triangle and, 53–4
　See also Drama Triangle
victim consciousness, 43–4
vulnerability
　men and, 217, 239–40
　Self-centered heart and, 165
　transformation and, 64, 178–9

waterfall of new beliefs
　exercise, 276–7
weighted pressure hold exercise, 222
White, Michael, 10
white supremacy, 31
Wolynn, Mark, 289
woundedness, 182
wounds, 182, 196–7, 198–9

Zen Mind, Beginner's Mind (Suzuki), 269

Also from Thornapple Press

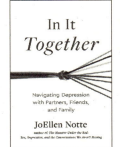

In It Together: Navigating Depression with Partners, Friends, and Family

JoEllen Notte

"Am I allowed to say I laughed and had so much fun reading about depression? Read this book and you'll feel seen—and you'll walk away with a real-life guide to helping loved ones without sacrificing your own mental health."

—Meredith Goldstein, Boston Globe Love Letters advice columnist, podcast host and author of *Can't Help Myself*

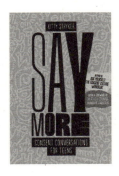

Say More: Consent Conversations for Teens

Kitty Stryker, with a foreword by Heather Corinna

"Don't be fooled into thinking this book is just for teens. It's terrific for adults too. In a rare combination of clarity and nuance, it's useful for everyone. And it's a joy to read."

—Dr. Betty Martin, author of *The Art of Receiving and Giving: the Wheel of Consent*

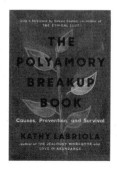

The Polyamory Breakup Book: Causes, Prevention, and Survival

Kathy Labriola, with a foreword by Dossie Easton

"*Mandatory reading for those considering an adventure into the world of consensual nonmonogamy.*"
—Ken Haslam, MD, founder of the Ken Haslam Polyamory Archives, the Kinsey Institute, Indiana University

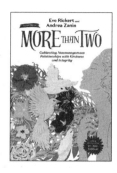

More Than Two, Second Edition: Cultivating Nonmonogamous Relationships with Kindness and Integrity

Eve Rickert with Andrea Zanin
Fully revised and updated second edition

"*In place of dominant and oppressive-for-so-many relationship norms, Eve Rickert and Andrea Zanin offer abundant possibilities that not only disrupt those norms, but that better meet the desires, needs, skills, and life conditions of the individual humans who are trying to love and relate as best we can in this challenging world.*"
—from the foreword by Dr. Kim TallBear, Professor and Canada Research Chair in Indigenous Peoples, Technoscience and Society at the University of Alberta and the author of *The Critical Polyamorist*.

ABOUT THE AUTHORS

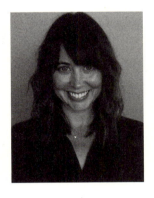

Jessica Fern is a psychotherapist, public speaker, and trauma and relationship expert. In her international private practice, Jessica works with individuals, couples and people in multiple-partner relationships who no longer want to be limited by their reactive patterns, cultural conditioning, insecure attachment styles and past traumas, helping them to embody new possibilities in life and love.

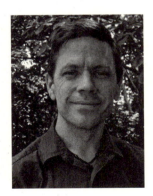

David Cooley is a professional restorative justice facilitator, diversity and privilege awareness trainer, and bilingual cultural broker. He is the creator of the Restorative Relationships Conversations model, a process that transforms interpersonal conflict into deeper connection, intimacy and repair. In his private practice, David specializes in working with non-monogamous and LGBTQ partnerships, incorporating a variety of modalities including trauma-informed care, attachment theory, somatic practices, narrative theory and mindfulness-based techniques.